FEAR FREE
Made Crystal Clear!

My Sounds Relieve Your Fears

DAWN CRYSTAL

outskirts
press

DEDICATION

This is for all those who suffer fear and anxiety and have lost hope. I want the world to know that there are alternative drug-free methods to relieve fear and anxiety that are safe, effective, and rapid. It takes some guidance and an open mind to obtain the possibilities of these non-traditional methods, including mine.

TABLE OF CONTENTS

FOREWORD

Some of what I present here I wrote for the Foreword for Dawn Crystal's first book, *PAIN FREE Made Crystal Clear!*, for which I served as editor/coach, too.

First, though, let me address fear. President Franklin Delano Roosevelt said, famously, "We have nothing to fear but fear itself." This has more than just a grain of truth, but it is clearly an over-statement. As the author of *The Gift of Fear* notes, there are times when it is wise to be fearful, when fear is sending us valuable signals to protect ourselves. However, we can also be unnecessarily fearful, which can depress us and make us make mistakes. Recently, I spent $10 at UnderstandMyself.com to take their psychological self-evaluation, allowing me to compare myself against thousands who have taken the same test. The 100-question test evaluates the user on five major traits (then broken down into two attributes each):

- Agreeableness (compassion and politeness)

- Conscientiousness (industriousness and orderliness)

- Extraversion (enthusiasm and assertiveness)

- Openness to experience (openness and intellect)

- Neuroticism (withdrawal and volatility).

As their names imply, the first four traits are positive and the last negative. Neuroticism is basically a sensitivity to negative emotions, including
worry and fear. Women tend to be higher in this than men, reporting
more unhappiness in general and initiating 70% of all divorces. To the
degree Dawn's techniques aid in reducing your fear and anxiety, you can
expect a general improvement in your attitudes and outcomes.

I "met" Dawn Crystal over the radio, Internet radio station WMAPradio.
com, where "WMAP" stands for "World's Most Amazing People," a
title for which she qualifies. During an extensive interview with host
KC Armstrong, she told how she developed her astonishing techniques
for relieving pain, by directing the internal energy of the person being
helped. She had previously been interviewed on ABC-TV, *The Today
Show, Dr. Oz,* etc. A vivacious and fluent guest, she also hosts her own
radio program from Hawaii on alternate Mondays.

Dawn is a pioneer of sound-energy relief of pain and anxiety. She
makes pain-relieving, fear-relieving sounds with her voice, a gift she
discovered as an adult. She has done this for over 20 years, with individuals or groups.

A health food store asked her to help "treat" customers…making her
sounds and blowing on their bodies. No medical claims were made.
Yet, many people reported feeling much better.

Subsequently, she found that many of her clients reported relief from
fear and anxiety. This book goes into that phenomenon, describing her
techniques and presenting testimonials to their effectiveness.

She now has a sophisticated web site, DawnCrystalHealing.com.
Dawn feels a Higher Power has guided her to go Internet, go global.
She started from nothing, "heart-guided."

Imagine a world free of fear and anxiety. Imagine if sources of pain could be fixed immediately, without drugs. Imagine being fear-free fast and easy. These are among Dawn's missions.

Who does she think should seek help? Anybody. Everybody. People who have tried everything else: holistic, natural, traditional. She's had success with a wide variety of fears and pains.

Sometimes she has discovered issues caused by unconscious influences. For example, she found that a client had been sexually abused as a child and didn't remember it.

What to make of all this? The testimonials are evidence that something beneficial is happening. We know that mind and body are interconnected. Hypnosis and auto-suggestion can produce dramatic changes, including pain and fear relief. Many medical successes are attributed to the "placebo effect," where belief in the likely efficacy of a cure helps produce a cure. Voodoo curses can cause the believers great harm. Human attraction, "animal magnetism," can make us feel better when we are ill or hurting. Faith healers have some surprising results, too.

A recent Internet neuroscience article discussed the successful use of sound to reduce anxiety:

[https://ideapod.com/neuroscientists-discover-song-reduces-anxiety-65-now-going-viral-listen/?utm_source=ideapod&utm_medium=email&utm_campaign=broadcast]

and the article stated that over 30% of people between 18 and 54 in the U.S. are affected by anxiety disorders. It has become the "number one mental health issue in North America." The article described a sound, a long song, that produced "a huge 65% reduction in people's overall anxiety levels." So, sound therapy is gaining acceptance.

A study by researchers at Denmark's Aarhus University, reported at neurosciencenews.com on 22 December 2016

https://neurosciencenews.com/dopamine-genetics-music-5806/,

found that "Sounds, such as music and noise, are capable of reliably affecting individuals' moods and emotions, possibly by regulating brain dopamine, a neurotransmitter strongly involved in emotional behavior and mood regulation… [it is] highly variable across individuals."

Discussing her techniques with Dawn, I found that her description of moving energy throughout the body and overcoming blockages resembled the techniques I learned years ago of auto-suggestion, self-hypnosis, in which progressive relaxation is produced by visualizing a warm, relaxing wave traveling through various parts of your body, starting with your feet. I have first-hand knowledge that such techniques worked for me, including relieving occasional tension headaches and facilitating falling asleep.

Those who would like to hear Dawn talk about herself and her techniques are invited to listen to this 25-minute interview done in August 2018, https://www.talkshoe.com/conf/summary/4977560.

I have been pleased to help get Dawn's story into print as her writing coach and editor. Another kind of personal change occurred: her energy and optimism have been infectious!

Douglas Winslow Cooper, Ph.D.
douglas@tingandi.com
WriteYourBookWithMe.com
Walden, NY
Autumn 2018

Acknowledgments

First, I thank my coach and editor, Douglas Winslow Cooper, Ph.D., without whom this book would not ever have been written.

My editor and I thank Cheryl C. Cohen, Director of Membership at the Greater Monroe [NY] Chamber of Commerce, for her skilled editorial assistance.

My pets – my dog, Hoku (Hawaiian for "star"), and my cats, Stitchy and Blacky – bring me daily joy and peace and deserve my gratitude. I can't imagine my life without them.

Disclaimer

The information in this book is not intended to be a replacement or substitute for medical advice. It does not diagnose, treat, or cure medical conditions. Please see a medical professional if you need help with such problems.

Preface

I wrote this book because I wanted everyone to know that there is hope for becoming fear-free, naturally, fast, easy, and effectively.

You should read this book if you are suffering from pain or anxiety or you know someone who is, and you or they have tried many different techniques without success to get relief.

As a gift to you, I am including this link to my introductory CD, which is directed toward relieving anxiety and insomnia:

https://drive.google.com/open?id=0B0lQ6PlNYe2AU21mQnpEd ThHekU

"Discover Sound Healing," normally sold for $20. I invite you to experience the soothing sounds channeled through my voice...to re-align yourself to your center. In as little as 20 minutes, you should feel peace through your physical body as your stress, anxiety, and worry disappear.

I am known by many for my healing vocals. I offer my sound healing sessions with a loving heart by phone and in person.

Dawn Crystal

DawnCrystalHealing@gmail.com

Maui, Hawaii

Autumn 2018

PROLOGUE: FEAR-FREE IN MINUTES

Out here in beautiful Maui, I have little to fear and much to celebrate, but fear plagues many of us. We hope to find the key to overcoming it. Amazon lists over 40,000 books, including 10,000 ebooks, on the topics, with titles like *Worry Less Live More, Beat Fear, Empower Your Fear, Fear, The Gift of Fear*, and *Feel the Fear...and Do Anyway*. No doubt, many of these are helpful. Here we will describe a new technique, pioneered by me, Dawn Crystal, that has helped many others overcome their fears and anxieties. We will also discuss some traditional approaches.

THE GIFT OF FEAR (de Becker, 2010)

Before discussing the relief of fear, I want to second Gavin de Becker's notion that sometimes fear is a positive factor in our lives, one to heed. If you are in a relationship with someone you fear, you would be well advised to get out of it. Spousal homicide, for example, is "the single most preventable serious crime in America." The book by de Becker and his free MOSAIC assessment system, available through his firm at Oprah's website, should be consulted. You are urged to follow this de Becker maxim: "Avoid being in the presence of someone who might do you harm."

Your intuition is a surprisingly good guide in this regard, as is a man's "gut feeling." Ignore this at your peril.

Now we can move on to less dire matters that frighten us. My website (DawnCrystalHealing.com) includes modules:

1 CLEARING RESISTANCE

2 CLEARING DOUBT & FEAR

3 CLEARING FEAR OF CHANGE

4 CLEARING FEAR OF GROWTH

5 CLEARING FEAR OF SUCCESS

6 CLEARING FEELING STUCK

7 GETTING CLEAR ON YOUR FUTURE

8 CLEARING CLUTTER

9 CLEARING FAMILY BLOCKS

10 DISCOVER THE ULTIMATE YOU!

11 GENERATE YOUR FUTURE SELF

12 TURNING BLOCKS INTO PROFITS

13 CLEARING SELF-SABOTAGE

14 CLEARING LACK OF SELF-WORTH

15 CLEARING YOUR FINANCIAL MESS

16 CLEARING FEAR OF SCARCITY

17 CLEARING THE BLOCKS TO WELCOMING & RECEIVING ABUNDANCE.

18 CLEARING FEAR OF LOSING A BELOVED PERSON OR PET

19 CLEARING FEAR OF DEATH.

The next chapters in this book explore each of these areas, along with clearing the fear of being seen.

Introduction: Overcoming My Fear-Filled Childhood

My childhood was filled with fear, almost from Day One.

My parents split when I was very young, before I even remember having two parents together. I must have been a year or two old, at most. Before they paired up, my mother and father, Bernice and Eugene, were neighbors in a middle-class area in Chicago in the 1960s, and my dad's family had come from Kansas.

Dad's folks owned an apartment house. My dad would be drinking while my mom was mowing the grass. They fell in love quickly. Their firstborn was Cindy, three years older than I. Then I came, and then Eugene, Jr., a year younger than I.

My mother had three sons from a former marriage almost twenty years before. In fact, Bernice and Eugene never did marry, so I was born "out of wedlock," "illegitimate."

My mother was a compulsive eater, perhaps due to her own early childhood lack of love. I was usually left alone or with an older sibling. I remember people telling me that I spent much time by myself. I sucked my thumb to reassure myself, which led to buck teeth, and some rejection due to my looks.

I shared a room with my younger brother. Two older brothers were in the room next door. They often raised a ruckus. My younger brother would huddle together with me, just as fearful as I was.

I had very few friends, as being from a welfare family with little money, I was viewed as somewhat undesirable. Some kind neighbors would invite us kids for meals, feeling sorry for us, but this did not make me feel accepted, especially as my older brothers were notorious for drinking, fighting, and drag racing deep into the night and early morning. I would look out the window at 2 a.m. and see my brothers being chased by cops. My mother ignored it.

After being kept up late up almost every night, I would have to go to school the next morning. I was poorly dressed, with hand-me-downs, unattractive, and a member of a family that most people disrespected. There was little in the way of child protection services in Chicago in the 1970s, little sympathy or help for me.

At school, especially in the early grades, my teachers would scream at me. Miss Rich and Mrs. Schorn would yell impatiently at me for being such a slow learner, and they would sit me in the corner, embarrassing me in front of the class.

"This is trash," one of them said as she tore up one of my third-grade papers. She did this in front of the whole class, shaming me. I turned deep red.

Kids can be vicious. Unattractive, with ill-fitting clothes, and buck teeth, I felt unwanted, disrespected, and disliked. Even in kindergarten, I got pushed around. I identified with Cinderella. Kids would actually physically fight with me after school. Reluctantly, I had to punch Jeanie, a classmate who was picking on me.

Daily, we went without supervision, my younger brother and I, throughout our whole childhood.

I got a paper route at age 9, delivering papers in the evenings, regardless of the weather. People looked critically at having this child selling papers at night.

One asked me, "Where's your mom?"

"I don't know."

"Why are you doing this?"

"I need to make money to buy myself some new clothes."

A few times, my father would invite me to go on vacations to northern Wisconsin with him and my younger brother; sometimes also my sister came, too. We'd go into the woods camping at his cabin. Mom was happy to have him pay for our food at that time, as he never gave her child support. So, this was a cost-saver for her.

We'd drive to the cabin in a fog of cigarette smoke, beer smell, dog odor. At the cabin, Dad would take us fishing, the best part of our trip. Dad drank Schlitz Malt Liquor, the booze he filled the refrigerator with.

After we'd return to the cabin, Dad would start lubricating himself, initially becoming a fairly happy drunk, then mutating to angry drunk, which made my brother and I go hide in the woods and hope the bears would leave us alone. At least the bears were sober! I was a nervous wreck and couldn't wait to get home. Fortunately, these "vacations" occurred only a few times.

My life seems a blur until I reached 14. A neighbor saw what I was going through and asked my mom if I could be taken under her wing, live with her. My mother agreed, and this saved my life, as this woman became like a benevolent aunt. She didn't want anything from this.

During this period, I lost several of my siblings–alcoholics and drug addicts. One brother died from a heroin overdose; another died from complications related to be being beaten severely in a bar. The hardest death was that of my younger brother, a year younger. He and his friends shot up heroin, He died at 16, severely addicted. He would beg to stay with me in my independent apartment, as the home situation was intolerable for him and for me. But he was a compulsive thief, stealing to get drugs. He died a slow, painful death from a staph infection that weakened his heart. These losses made me really think about life. I also think this made me go into law enforcement later. I had a drive to help other people and improve society.

Eventually, I graduated from high school. While there, I started dating a guy in the school band. I had met him when I was 14. Lee was Southern. I liked him a lot, but I did not know what love was like, as I never experienced it from my family. Lee and I got into sex too young, leading to my having a miscarriage at 16. I dated him for nine years. into my early twenties. Frankly, I guess he was using me for sex.

I became pregnant again in my teens, and my mother wanted me to keep it, but Lee did not, so I got an abortion.

I worked as a hostess at IHOP at 16 and was happy that I could buy myself some decent clothes. After graduation from high school, I became a store manager at Dunkin' Donuts.

That relationship with Lee fizzled out in my early 20s.

I moved to a job at a plastics company. Next, Randy, 15 years older than I, dated me. He was attracted to me but could not love me. I figured that out, slowly. Randy and I were together into my late 20s. Somehow, I finally realized this was not for me.

My dad worked in a blue-collar sanitation job for the City of Chicago. His bragging about the benefits of that City job encouraged me to take the test for the Chicago Police Department. I passed. This helped me get out of the plastics company and out of that toxic, draining relationship with Randy.

I spent six months at the Police Academy. I had never shot a gun before, and I was nearly petrified at first. I would stand on the range, with my arms shaking and my body shivering. Somehow (divine intervention?), I passed that test. The written test, because I had a learning disability, I spent more time to study for. They ran us seemingly for hours. I was the fastest runner of the female class in the training group, probably from the fleeing I did while younger. I got my choice of districts in Chicago and took one not too far from my home.

The cop job was a big pay upgrade in my life. I did about five years on the force. My new partner and I patrolled Wrigley Field and another park. From all those hours patrolling together and talking in the squad car, I slowly bonded with my squad-car partner, Steve, a divorced man, soft-spoken, undemanding, one who would not take advantage of me. We married and bought a condo together. Unfortunately, to improve his vision, Steve chose to get a pair of Lasik eye operations, a relatively recent technology which ended up blinding him. This destroyed all the things we could do together, HIs career was ruined, and he had negligible disability benefits. I ended up leaving the police department to help care for him.

We moved to Pennsylvania, bought a condo with the results of a small lawsuit we won. We lived near Lake Erie. He started drinking, and our marriage fell apart. We got a divorce. Steve split our assets with me, allowing me to start a business, a tanning salon. I had no business background, having to learn by doing.

Enter the next significant other person: "Jim" (not his name), a handsome, macho body-builder tanning client caught my eye, way too soon after my divorce. Turns out he was a gigolo, living off women, and he started living off me at my apartment almost right after I met him.

We married soon. He changed drastically right after. He would go to bars on his motorcycle, ignoring me.

I was obviously "Looking for love in all the wrong places."

You and I know motorcycles are dangerous. Not too long after marrying him, I got a call from a hospital, "Your husband has been in a major motorcycle accident."

He spent months in the intensive care ward, while I tried to care for him and also run a business.

This was the lowest time of my life. Nothing was working out for me. I was not sharing love, just being used.

"Aren't you ever going to work?" I asked this drinker. Apparently not.

I got a divorce.

The tanning business fizzled, and I was losing money while my condo was losing value. In fact, I went bankrupt. At this low point, I gave away whatever I had left and moved, severing all ties. He got the house, and I got a one-way ticket to the Hawaiian Islands, following my heart and a magazine ad that said, "Go to the Sun!"

With two bags of clothes, I flew to Hawaii. It looked good in a magazine. I did not tell the others. Just dropped my stuff, taking my last seven hundred dollars to Oahu, along with some jewelry.

I could not afford an apartment. I got a ten-year-old Rent-a-Wreck car and lived out of it for many months. This became my new island home.

Was I crazy to give up everything I had left behind?

No, I got an energy boost from being on Oahu.

Then I got a job in a jewelry store, part-time, allowing me to get food, like dollar meals at McDonald's. I'd bathe by sneaking into hotel resort pools or using the public showers at the beach. I occasionally pawned my jewelry to keep my car going.

The Hawaiian police wanted vagrants to keep moving, and that included me. They wanted us off the streets. One place they did not push us from was parking by the beach, where I went to save on gas money, by not having to move my car so much.

Worried that I was crazy, I was sitting on the beach, humming along, and sounds were coming through my voice. I was making sounds that got stronger and stronger, helping me feel better. I was self-medicating with sound! I did this for hours, stone sober, as I have never been on drugs.

"What are you doing, lady?" a curious beach-goer asked.

"I'm making sounds that help me."

"Can I stay and listen?"

"Yes."

"Your sounds are making me feel better, too."

Some people would sit with me for hours. This was unusual back at that time, as spirituality was generally considered "weird," "voodoo."

In fact, this making of healthful sounds was my God-given gift.

A woman who ran a spa told her boss about me, and they decided to ask me to go into the spa and do nighttime sessions by a luau. My non-contact sound sessions appealed to her and to her clients.

"Whatever money you make," she offered, "I'll give you half."

This started out slowly and then picked up. People were puzzled by it but pleased with the results. I made the sounds, sometimes blowing on people's bodies, and did some intuitive readings. We did this for months. I was making money.

Next, local vitamin stores, health food stores, had me come with a table, a chair, and a tip jar. I released blockages for their customers, who then started requesting my phone number. Soon, I could afford a cell phone. I tried doing phone sessions, and they worked. As word spread, I was able to start a web site. Hawaii is a bit like a small town in that the word spread. My web site started taking off.

My intuitive work led to a job on Maui, to supplement my security job with hotels (recall my police experience). I was able to afford to get my dog in Pennsylvania to join me on the island. Sadly, this sweetie lived only two more years. Later, another dog, Hoku, now eight years old, joined me when he was just a little puppy.

Now my life has taken off, and things are better than I could have imagined.

I have fine-tuned my gift, allowing me to work globally, by phone or Skype, and I get requests even to do sessions by phone with patients of certain doctors.

Having been through so many hardships, I have conquered my fears. I now enjoy helping others conquer theirs as well.

Chapter 1

CLEARING RESISTANCE

SOMETIMES WE WANT to do something and yet we cannot get ourselves to do it. Our energy is blocked. We probably have not fully convinced ourselves that we can do it.

In psychotherapy, resistance to therapy surprisingly strengthens as we get closer to the main issue.

With my sound sessions, we try another way around the blockage.

Many people come to me with their fears, such as a fear of not having enough money. I often detect a below-conscious fear of receiving benefits. Perhaps they do not feel worthy. Our egos are strange about such topics. They need to be made more receptive, less resisting.

The problem may start with ideas that they learned from their parents, perhaps that they only deserve a little, not a lot, not more than what they "need." Maybe they won't pursue a certain career or opportunity because they don't think it will pay enough to support them or they don't see the value in it right away.

One kind of resistance is being unfamiliar with non-traditional healing. They don't know what to expect, and perhaps they are not sure I'm the right person, though they have taken the chance to work with me.

Some think there is only one way a goal can be reached, and they rule out other ways that might be even more successful. They need to see a path to the goal or, even better, have faith that they can get there on their own. They need to be in a more receptive state, an openness to other alternatives than they are currently considering, heeding the true guidance they can obtain from their heart chakra area. That guidance will produce an "aha!" or "yes!" response when they are on the right track, following the right path. This response will guide them in the right direction.

Here are some excerpts from a typical session:

The client says, "I have resistance. I can't get past this level in my life."

To help, I produce sound frequencies that somehow seem appropriate for them, almost "sounds of their souls." Their speech slows down. Their breathing deepens. They relax. For the rest of the 30-minute sessions, I work with them, following my gift.

I'll often ask, "Do you know what you are resisting?"

"More love. More money. I don't know where it is coming from."

I vocalize more, and they go into a deeper state of relaxation.

I find such resistance often has begun even before the age of six. The family story contributes to this, and the children, like sponges, absorb the family belief system. Sometimes, the source of the belief system is not the family but another person significant in the life of the growing child.

As we age, we attract some influences unconsciously. We may resist things we want, thinking we are not worthy or that they are somehow to be feared.

During our sessions, we will go into a silent period, and I am tuning into their unconscious mind, showing me which way to go with the person.

"What don't you like about your life situation?" I'll ask.

They begin to identify what they do not like. I sense a movement of energy. I have a built-in sense of how they are responding. That is almost a psychological GPS to help me find their problem quickly.

"How do you feel now?"

"I feel great."

"You'll find that this feeling will continue after our call. You'll find that your resistance has decreased and continues to do so for days or even weeks. Take a deep breath. How do you feel now?"

"Much more peaceful. My internal resistance energy seems to have cleared. I don't feel that heavy burden I felt before the call."

Often, I will hear from clients telling me that the problem situations have cleared up and new opportunities have come into their lives. Some have been so good as to write testimonials (see some toward the back of this book).

Chapter 2

CLEARING DOUBT & FEAR

ONE WAY TO reduce doubt is to get more information. We can ask others who have useful knowledge or find ourselves some useful books and articles. At some point, we have to stop collecting information and make a decision that comes down on one side or the other of the issue bugging us.

Some "information" is hidden within us, perhaps as intuition or as feelings. Thinking and re-thinking may not get us the answer we seek. I believe my sound sessions help us tap the inner voices that reason alone cannot reach.

Until you have resolved your doubts, it is quite logical to have a fear of going forward. As your psychological energy dissolves your doubt and fear, you are able to progress.

Many people have a mental/emotional block of doubt and fear. It gets in the way of their improving things, accessing new opportunities. I can hear it in their voices. In my sessions, I am clearing the unconscious blocks with their help.

For example, often they want more wealth. They don't know how to break through their blocks, conscious or unconscious, to manifest it.

I start by asking about their childhoods. Wealthy? Poor? Usually, they felt poor, their parents often complaining about money, "Money doesn't grow on trees." This puts doubt and fear into their subconscious.

"What do you want to work on today?" I asked.

Jean, from France, an affluent, confident businesswoman, spoke of making great deals, but then having her ideas stolen by others who then grab her customers. In romantic relationships, she found the same: the relationship doesn't last; it breaks up after a while.

I said to Jean, "Tell me about growing up."

Her mother had real anxiety issues and was taking numerous medicines. I could tell that Jean is an unusually empathic person, and she readily picked up her mother's angst. Furthermore, she was not getting reassurance from her mother, even while Jean was trying to help her.

Unfortunately, Jean had taken on much of her mother's doubt and fears.

Once she relaxed, I performed a deep clearing of her conscious mind.

"Jean, what don't you like about your life now? Is your mother still alive? Would you like to break through this barrier?"

"Yes. Nothing has seemed to work out for me."

"Think about your businesses and your romantic relationships while I start to move your energy."

Then I made my healing sounds to clear her unconscious mind.

"How do you feel now?"

"I don't feel quite so blocked."

I did more energy moving and some visualization.

We returned to the topic of her mother. "I'm going to clear your past interaction with your mother."

Jean started crying.

"You are holding much of your mom's fears in your solar plexus. This helps explain your constipation problems."

"My stomach feels lighter now."

"You were storing this blocked energy in your stomach area. Now, breathe deeply."

Her crying stopped.

"Jean, how do you feel now that we did the clearing?"

"I feel relieved. My stomach no longer has the feeling of a cement block. I hear it, too. My heart also seems different."

"This is what has been blocking you. In a few weeks, send me an email about your progress."

She did just that. In a few weeks, she reported that things were changing for her for the better. She was getting more clients, feeling physically better, even less constipated. She was surprised that this all came from one 30-minute session, and she had a second session with me.

Most of the problems my clients have come from fear, fear that has been put into them when they were young. Children are like sponges, absorbing thoughts readily, so we have to be careful what we tell them.

Chapter 3

CLEARING FEAR OF CHANGE

THERE IS NOTHING irrational about fearing change. You understand, or think you do, the situation you are in at present. Change will bring a new situation with new benefits and losses, and it is hard to determine whether you will be better off.

When you can decide whether or not to institute the change, you can listen to your thoughts and your emotions and decide what course to take.

When you do not control the change, then you must find out how to adapt to it. Some adaptation will be by changing your behavior and your thoughts about the new situation. Some will come from modifying your emotions, re-directing your psychological energy. Here is an area in which my sound techniques are likely to be most effective.

This is a very common situation. People want change on one level and

fear it on another. The change might be physical, financial, occupa-
tional, or a family situation. Often, the adult side is at odds with the
child side; the inner child, their unconscious mind, is most resistant to
change.

One lady, Beth, was in a stifling relationship, and she wanted to change.
She scheduled a 30-minute phone session.

"What do you want to work on, Beth?"

"My marriage, for the first half of our 25 years, it was wonderful. Then
he got injured, and even though he had physical therapy, he became
quite changed…angry and controlling."

I worked only with Beth, not with her husband.

"Beth, you did the right thing to support him as you did when he was
hurt, but this is much too long to put up with a controlling person, an
anti-social person. He is turning you into a hermit, and the love has
been lost between you two."

"I've given 100%, but it is not being appreciated. I have more life left
in me! I want to get out into the world and contribute, as I used to do,
like reading to children and writing. I want a change."

"You clearly want to change, and by calling me, you indicated you are
ready to do it. Can I scan your energy?" She agreed to allow me to do
so.

A thirty-minute session led to discovering that, as she was growing
up, her father had similar tendencies to those of her husband; he had
been controlling, somewhat abusive to the six kids. Her mother was to
cater to him. He was cold to the children. Beth was trying to get his

love; sadly, her dad had himself been raised in a harsh environment. He provided for their needs but did not show them love. Once grown, she looked for love from other men, without success. The romantic relationships would start well, but soon decline. They would fizzle out. Then she met "John," initially charming. They fell in love, married. Then an accident changed him, made him much more controlling, angry, verbally abusive.

"Is there something you can do to keep me from attracting this kind of situation?"

I went into her child mind, clearing it with sound, with her permission. Told her she was OK as she is, and she can be independent if she needs to be.

"Yes, I'd like to be an author and give more to the outside world."

I could see that her inner child feared abandonment, but I reassured her that she would not grow old and lonely. I told her she did not need another person's love. We did an additional 30 minutes to clear up the unconscious energy from her childhood. I then moved to higher frequency energies, to combat this "battered-wife syndrome."

"We've worked almost an hour; how do you feel?"

"Much lighter, freer, with a spring in my step, ready to do something."

I gave her some suggestions, practical ones, about joining with people in the world outside her marriage. "Visualize your life as you want it, not what you don't want. Picture it as a pleasant movie. You need to start journaling, describing the life you want. How do you want your life re-made, Beth?"

                    FEAR FREE MADE CRYSTAL CLEAR!

"I've worked with others, spending thousands of dollars, making little progress. I've been very pleased with you, and I want to book another session."

About a month later, we had another session.

"How are you doing, Beth?"

"I've made more change in the past three weeks than I made in all my prior life. I'm networking with some very creative and helpful ladies. They are helping me to help children. Journaling has gotten me prepared to write my first book. Even my husband sees the change. I gave him an ultimatum for the first time, and he respected it. He is supportive now, and said before he thought we were both dying, but my new energy, my being happy has helped him. Just that short session not only helped me but has gotten him at least to go out on the porch, to do some reading. I was given the courage to change, and this has been good for both me and him. He is picking up on my positive new energy. Your work has been miraculous, and more people need to know about you."

It is never too late for us to make changes in our lives. We are co-creators of our reality, and we must focus on what we want, bringing positive new energy through visualization, doing it consistently to make changes in our lives. We will then become more aware of many small opportunities we might have overlooked before. Baby steps will become giant leaps.

Chapter 4

CLEARING FEAR OF GROWTH

FEAR OF GROWTH is a form of fear of change, but a particularly unfortunate form, as growth often offers real benefits and few disadvantages. Again, a rational analysis of the positive and negative elements is valuable, and you are likely to conclude that the growth will be beneficial overall.

Still, you may have a remaining fear, an emotional reluctance, and you want to re-direct your energy into overcoming this, so that you can get the benefits of growth. A session that re-directs your energy using the sound techniques may be all that's needed to overcome this fear.

Recently, I started working with Whitney, a thirty-something phone client who found out about me through my telesummit show, and she bought a program that included a 30-minute phone session with me.

The first session had her express her complaints about how her life was stagnating, very different from the life she had some half-dozen years before. Having turned 30, she found that things slowed down, and she became less sociable.

I asked Whitney, "What has changed from your twenties to your thirties?"

"I don't know. I was in a relationship for about three years, at first a wonderful relationship, until he started becoming very controlling, knocking down my self-esteem."

"That's understandable. You unconsciously allowed this person to harm you."

"That has been a pattern with me. I become needy, and the person and I drift apart. He becomes unresponsive."

"Seems a pattern with you. Let's see why."

"Yes, and I'm afraid to meet new people, I fear this rejection will happen."

I had a sense about how this started, "Tell me about your childhood."

"I had a pretty traumatic childhood. At age two, I was with my folks on a boat on Lake Huron, and the boat capsized, tossing us all in the water, and my mother and two brothers drowned. Three years later, Dad got into another relationship with a woman, withdrawing his love from me. The new woman did not warm up to me, and she had her own children. I felt there was something wrong with me, unworthy. I tried hard at everything, to get my dad's praise and attention. I was an overachiever, in the classroom and at sports, but he never really showed me love. Marrying that second women kept him separated from me."

"This is quite understandable. You were not being given the love that every child needs and should expect. This trauma can get stored within ourselves. We are going to try to release that traumatic energy. Picture a light over your head, a divine light. Go back to being age two."

Whitney started crying.

I was making my soothing sounds, and then I told her, "Surrender any hurt that you feel. Move that energy out of your body."

We then discussed her later life. Still, she was feeling ignored.

"Picture the energy moving away from your stomach. Take some deep breaths."

She did that.

"You have not gotten the love you deserved. You are looking for it now. The people you are seeing are sensing and mirroring your neediness."

She was very nervous.

"You have to know that you don't have to over-achieve to be worthy, to be noticed. You are attracting the wrong people. Are you able to move forward with your life? To move to another part of the country, where you have a new job offer?"

"I want to do that, but I fear change."

"Whitney, I think you need to take this job and relocate."

"I wanted to do that, but I was afraid to say yes. Now I feel like I could do it."

"You were stuck before, but now things are shifting for you."

"Yes, I was afraid, but I am going to see if the job is still available. I'll have another session with you, and I will let you know."

A month went by.

"Hi, Whitney, how is it going? "

"The dam has broken free, and I have felt very changed, and I contacted them about the job, and I am flying across the country from Oregon to DC to interview. I am going to sell my house and relocate."

She was clearly excited, "My life is moving forward, and I am no longer afraid of the change. I did not know before that the wounds as a child were holding me back. Now I see that, and I feel free from that. I am grateful for your help, which has changed my life."

She did end up getting the job she wanted and moving to Washington, DC, and she sold her house at a decent price.

Sometimes we reach a stage in our lives where we are blocked, often due to painful experiences from our childhood. If we can release the pain, we can move forward. In Whitney's case, it allowed her to rewrite the script for her life, move to a new location, and find the happiness that had been denied her.

Chapter 5

CLEARING FEAR OF SUCCESS

WHY WOULD YOU fear success? In an article on this topic [https://99u. adobe.com/articles/14347/are-you-subconsciously-afraid-of-success] Mark McGuinness listed the following:

1. **Fear of Not Coping with Success**. Success is usually more complicated than failure, and it puts you in positions you are not familiar with.

2. **Fear of Selling Out**. You are not sure that you will preserve your integrity, that you won't be seen by others as having traded important values for money or fame.

3. **Fear of Becoming Someone Else**. You will join a new peer group, and to some degree you will start to absorb their values and behavior. Friends and family may not like this. Your views may change, too, as "where you stand depends on where you sit," the adage goes.

Some of our fears are generated by childhood experiences that make us afraid of new situations, including success. You can handle such issues by analysis, but sometimes you may need to approach them through the emotional/energy channels reached by sound-based intervention.

"Jim" is a doctor. A good person, a chiropractor. I needed his chiropractic help, but after a couple of sessions, I realized he was harming himself with his thinking. When I went into Jim's office for some holistic work, the first impression I had was that the place was old-fashioned, outdated, almost industrial. No curb appeal. I wanted some physical help and I was not being judgmental, but I did notice these things. The wallpaper was outdated, and the curtains were iffy, and he seemed to have the rest of his home on the other side of them. Even the bathroom was shabby.

I greeted him with, "I have heard you are very good at natural chiropractic work. I'd like some balancing and some body work, a light treatment."

As he worked with me, I realized he was quite good. I wondered why he did not have a better-looking set-up. I thought I'd go back again. I had some injuries from accidents while I was a police officer. He did make me feel better.

The second appointment, I still was aware of the run-down appearance of his office. Although I tried not to judge him by it, the set-up made me less confident of his abilities. We discussed our childhoods. He had grown up, as I did, with an abusive, alcoholic father. We shared this. The session went well, physically and emotionally.

I had bought a package of five sessions. The third one went fine. We did some more body work. He helped me. I felt rapport with Jim, as he seemed to have a good heart. We developed a friendship of sorts.

I asked him, "Are you married? Have kids?"

"No, I never married. I hope to find the love of my life, but I've had trauma, as you have."

"You seem successful, and I would think you'd have a big following. You've got I diplomas from impressive places. Still, your car is old, and I fear you are not having the success you deserve."

Frankly, the people in his waiting room looked like they had little money.

"Jim, do you do some of your work for free?"

"Yes, or for cash. I just seem to have gravitated to this, giving others a break."

"You seem to be somewhat lacking in office help."

Jim frowned, "Yes, I have a helper, but we are just getting by."

"Are you prospering?"

"No."

"Well, I'd be happy to help you with my gift," I offered.

"That would be good. Money never stays with me. Women who see my set-up decide they don't want to date me."

I volunteered that we could discuss toxic patterns the next time I came.

Pleased, Jim said, "We can exchange services, gifts to each other."

                    FEAR FREE MADE CRYSTAL CLEAR!

Next session, I gave him some sound-clearing. "I feel you have some blocks here. You have a fine reputation, but you are scraping by in terms of money."

"I agree, I don't know why I am not prospering, not thriving."

Growing up, Jim was abused by his father, screaming at him at the top of his lungs. It was fight-or-flight, and he lost much of his hearing as a child. He was bullied, as I was, at school.

"It is understandable that you are lacking confidence," I said.

"In school, once I started weight-lifting, building myself up, playing on the football team, girls showed new interest in me."

Still, even now he was not really advertising his services.

"Imagine you are looking at the kids who once beat you up and at your father and others who did not treat you well." I made some clearing sounds. He imagined his father coming and shouting. I moved that energy, cleared it out.

"You're stuck in a pattern of playing it small, not being seen. I am releasing energy connected with this."

Jim smiled, "Wow, let's wait another day to work on you."

I grounded him before I left. He had been crying while I worked.

"You are looking calmer, and I think we released some blockage that was holding you back."

"I agree, I feel you have released some blockages."

He actually paid me. I thanked him.

A week later, I was there to get fixed, to get another treatment. "Jim, how are you doing?"

"Something has changed. I had felt stuck, afraid to be myself, to move forward. Now I am willing to charge for my services, and I am advertising more. I am charging or asking for a donation, which I did not do before, as though I did not feel I was worthy of being paid. I'm going to trade in my old car for something newer. I am motivated to take action."

He hadn't had a picture of himself as a success, and he felt not worthy of it, as his father had told him he would be a failure and the school kids would chase him home.

Despite his training and expertise, he did not feel he deserved success, and my sounds and advice helped remove him from this mental box to see what was really happening to him.

I find that sometimes a professional must go to another professional to get expert treatment. Jim was grateful for my help, and I for his.

Chapter 6

CLEARING FEELING STUCK

DO OR NOT do? Go or not go? You are stuck. Undecided. At a standstill. Recently, Allie Green wrote a fine piece [https://www.mindbodygreen.com/articles/5-things-to-do-if-youre-feeling-stuck-in-life] giving advice on becoming unstuck:

1. **Listen to Your Body.** Find a quiet place and quiet time and think about the alternatives you are confronting and see how your body feels when you think about each. You may learn much.

2. **Pay Attention to Your Thoughts**. We generally become what we think we can be, so we have to control our thoughts to influence our future. Identify false negativities and detect areas that legitimately need improvement. Give yourself the benefit of a positive mantra, such as "I AM enough!"

3. **Engage in Wanderlust.** Do something different. Go somewhere you don't usually go. Shake up the daily pattern a bit. The new experiences promote new thoughts. You might even turn off your cell phone awhile!

4. **Look for Signs from the Universe.** What? Well, we receive zillions of impressions daily and only some of them we notice. Why do we notice some and not others? Perhaps because they resonate with something inside us. Inspiration comes when we make the connections with awareness. Synchronicity succeeds!

5. **Share Your Stuckness.** Yes, fessing up to it, especially to someone important to you, someone whose advice your value, can get you help and can open your mind. They may have or help generate some valuable insights.

These primarily rational/analytical approaches to being stuck have their value, but it is likely that "stuck" is another way of saying your energy is blocked, which is where my sound techniques can be beneficial.

Wanting to change and feeling stuck is common. It becomes a habit. As we mature, we add habits that are hard to change. We need to shake things up a little. One client, a mid-Westerner, bought one of my 30-minute sessions: Pat was from Kansas, married many years, in the same house for 20-plus years, raising her five kids there, with a happy 40-year marriage to her childhood sweetheart.

"I feel my life is kind of ending now. I have low energy, having gained some twenty pounds. I love my husband, but I just feel trapped, stagnant. The house needs fixing up, but I don't have the energy to do it, and I want to move to another part of the state. I'm stuck. I don't want to invest more into this house."

"Pat, let's explore why you don't want to renovate the house and move."

Turned out that she had a strong belief that she should keep the house that had belonged to her parents. This was something she thought her family wanted her to do, as she had inherited it.

"Pat, you told me your parents told you to do whatever you want with the house, but you are reluctant to sell it."

"My siblings were less responsible than I. My parents always praised me for that. They gave me this house almost as a reward for doing well and being responsible. They are now gone, yet I feel their influence."

"Maybe we can get you beyond feeling stuck. Look around at other homes and imagine yourself living there."

"Yes, this is from my childhood, feeling I must please my dead parents by keeping the house."

I had her focus on what she did not like about the current situation, including the house, while we had a few minutes of silence. I then cleared her energy, which was blocked throughout her body, trapped just like she felt she was.

"I'm feeling I can breathe again."

I worked on moving her energy.

"How do you feel now?"

"More alive, with more energy, and a cloud over my head has been lifted."

"Could you start looking around to find a more manageable living situation?"

"Yes, a smaller house, with less property, and less upkeep."

"Good, look at new places daily; check them out."

"I'm going to do that. I'm newly motivated. I will also schedule another session with you."

We scheduled another appointment for two weeks later.

"Pat, how is everything going? Are you still stuck?"

"Oh, my God, as soon as I got off the phone, I looked into a real estate magazine, found a property, a senior home, and my husband and I looked at it. It was a single-family home in a senior community, a house with minimal upkeep, and it even had a clubhouse and swimming pool. I love swimming, and can swim there year-round, as the pool is heated. We are putting our house up for sale, and we have already gotten inquiries, especially from people interested in the land, regardless of the condition of the house. We will move to this senior community and be confident we can sell the house and land. Thank you so much. I'll update you. I'm not feeling stuck but energized. We've put a down-payment on the house. Thanks so much."

A month and a half later, she emailed me that she sold the house in a couple of weeks, as is, and the next place is being built.

Trusting her heart had led Pat to new opportunities and to a new life.

Chapter 7

Getting Clear On Your Future

THINK BACK SEVERAL years or several decades in your life. What would you have predicted for yourself? How close to correct would you have been? I find that my big changes were often big surprises. That means we probably cannot predict our future now, either.

Your future will be determined by things out of your control and things you can control, and you want to pay attention to the latter. Acquire knowledge, be prudent with money, take care of your health, nurture beneficial relationships, spend your time wisely…these steps will help shape what is to come.

Some of your concern for the future can be relieved by my techniques, and your improved mood and enhanced energy will help you shape better outcomes.

I helped a lady, Roseanne, who contacted me. She got one of my programs I sell on my telesummit. We had a 30-minute session.

"What's going on? What do you want to change?"

She was depressed, talking fast, feeling trapped. "For many years I've been living in partial ownership of a house with my aunt. My life feels stuck. The house needs repair. I'd need 20 thousand dollars to do it that I don't have. My life is not going anywhere. I'm feeling trapped, dying."

"What do you do for a living?"

"I'm on disability. I can't drive. I have trouble seeing. I must depend on others. I'm only 55. I have no hobbies."

"What do you want from our session?"

"I need change. I've had some dead-end relationships after I inherited part of a house. My aunt and I are stuck."

"What can we change?"

"I want to change my living situation, which has been negative ever since my mother died."

I started to move her energy. She was blocked. She did need to sell her house.

"I don't know how to do it. My aunt can't afford to pay me her share, her half."

I told her she needed legal advice that I could not give. I was sure she could find a way to sell the house and share the money from it. "You need to find an expert to help you, instead of waiting for your aunt to pass away. Secondly, you need to become more outgoing. Do you have a hobby that you could warm up again?"

                                    FEAR FREE MADE CRYSTAL CLEAR!

"I used to write. I never wrote a book, but I really want to."

I told Roseanne, "Journaling every day would be a good start to writing again."

She replied, "I used to write articles for a local newspaper, but I got downsized."

"Other publications might want you."

"There's a ladies' club publication that won't pay but wants help."

"That would get you going, get you out of the house. Any other passions?"

"I love animals!"

"Humane societies need help, and some even pay."

She brightened up. "Neighbors have told me this, too, but it is stronger coming from you."

"Yes. You've got to get your life going again."

"I'll check with a realtor about the house, and maybe we can sell it as is, and I could pay off my aunt."

She was getting to be more positive. I told her, "Write down in your daily journal what you want in your life. Do some visualization about what you want, not what you fear."

"No one has told me that before."

"We'll do some energy work now. Energy blocks have been holding you back. When we're done, you'll see better how to make some changes for your future."

I did some clearing and moving of her energy, especially moving the negative energy emotions about her aunt and her house. A few minutes went by.

"How do you feel now?"

"Much better. I feel I am getting off the hamster wheel I've been on."

I worked to relieve her negative energy. I moved her energy to ground her.

"Oh, my gosh, I feel I can actually think! I was feeling stuck and lonely, and I thought I couldn't change my future. Now, I am ready to get some questions answered by someone who knows about real estate."

"Sure, you might sell it for a profit, and find yourself a place to live on your own."

"I'm feeling excited, even giddy."

She booked another session for about a month later.

I began that session, "How are you doing today?"

"Believe it or not, my life has started to change. I've looked through magazines and newspapers and found realtors who know my area and who think I can get a lot of money for my house, much more than I expected. I feel there's some hope. I can pay off my aunt and live on my own. I'm going to get myself a condo. I joined a ladies' club, and I'm the writer for the club bulletin, and they are paying me to be the club secretary!"

FEAR FREE MADE CRYSTAL CLEAR!

While she was growing up, Roseanne's family had been depressing. She had taken on most of her mom's sadness, because Roseanne herself was quite empathetic, absorbing her family's pain.

It was clear Roseanne had gotten renewed hope for her future, a future that would involve real changes. Our energy movement sessions helped raise her optimism, and she acquired an eagerness for a changed life, including a possible romance.

"I'm feeling so much more light, happy. Now I realize I had taken on my mom's depression."

She left, thanking me, telling me her life had been changed, her future resolved.

I find that many of my clients don't think enough about what they want. Even a bit of visualization can help them, and moving and discarding negative energy thoughts helps make room for what they do want.

Our sound-energy sessions provide opportunities for change to better futures. Journaling daily helps as well, picturing what an ideal life should be like. Working on their own lives after our sessions pays real dividends. My clients co-create their own success.

Chapter 8

CLEARING CLUTTER

A WILDLY SUCCESSFUL book on cleaning up one's household clutter is Marie Kondo's *The Life-changing Magic of Tidying Up: The Japanese Art of Decluttering and Organizing*. She has you organize by categories and keep only what "sparks joy." Her followers have almost cult-like devotion.

Well, perhaps you are not ready to go whole-hog into clearing clutter, and in fact, you might want to clear clutter in your brain rather than in your living room. You may want to learn how to be comfortable in your clutter or you may need an energy boost before you tackle it. For this, we have a "sound solution."

"Susan" gradually became a hoarder. Her neighbor watched as things started to pile up in and around Susan's home: a half-dozen dogs, 13 cats, a big pooper of a land turtle, a giant bird house with ten screeching parrots, a pen full of chickens, a caged dog who cried and barked incessantly, plus stuff in the carport, from floor to ceiling…furniture, massive bags of pet food, lots of plastic coverings.

As if that were not enough, Susan and her husband boarded dogs in their three-bedroom home. Talk about a full house!

Aware of Susan's condition, a mutual friend had put us together. Susan wanted help, using my holistic counseling service. Susan had heard many success stories and was eager to change.

We had a 30-minute phone session.

"Hi, Susan, how are you doing? This is Dawn Crystal; a friend said that you might want me to help you to get unstuck."

"I'm am stuck! I'm depressed. I moved from a bigger house to this one, and the contents are overwhelming me. Plus, I've got lots of animals. Even so, something is missing in my life."

"How long have you lived this way?"

"All my life it seems."

"What else would you like to do?"

"Well, my husband uses the birds for photography. Someone has to take care of them. I used to dress up and go to a fine office job as an office manager, but the business closed down, and I became a stay-at-home mom, and I took care of my elderly father, too."

I did some sound therapy with her, then I asked her, "Would you want to get a part-time job?"

"I've tried. They look at me as old, and they ask for computer skills I don't have.'

"It might be different now," I offered, "there are new hotels going up, and the new places are hiring now and willing to take on part-time workers and even give them some training."

She surprised me, "OK. I'll go on-line to apply."

We went back to my sound-session, "Let's do some energy-clearing...."

After we finished, Susan seemed energized, "I am going to take some action steps, because I have been feeling I am dying."

A few weeks later, we later had another session.

"How have you doing now, Susan?"

"I had two interviews, then I did a third one at a new hotel, and they hired me! I start part-time, after their orientation program. I cannot believe that I could have stayed stuck in my old situation. I thought I wasn't marketable, but in fact my office experience was just what they were looking for. Frankly, I feel lighter and not so grumpy. I'm so glad my friend put you and me together. I am donating some of my stuff to the less fortunate, and the house already seems more open, less cluttered."

In fact, I had recently seen a giant U-Haul truck leave her house.

If you are feeling stuck and stagnated, look around at what is going on and get rid of those dust-collectors; donate them or sell them. You'll find you feel better, and you will help others who need just what you have too much of. It feels nice to make a difference in the lives of others. You'll get an energy boost as you reduce the clutter that gets in your way and on your nerves.

                    FEAR FREE MADE CRYSTAL CLEAR!

Chapter 9

CLEARING FAMILY BLOCKS

MELANIE PINOLA RECENTLY wrote a valuable article, "Top 10 Family Issues You Can Overcome," [https://lifehacker.com/top-10-family-issues-you-can-overcome-1674901208]. Here is a list of her issues and a brief summary of her approaches:

1. **Being Far from Your Family.** Use technology where possible to increase the number and depth of your communication with them. Visit often, if you can.

2. **Being too Close to Family.** There is some wisdom in the saying, "Absence makes the heart grow fonder." More likely, we seek a golden mean. Too close can produce friction. Too far produces alienation. Decide on boundaries and stick to them.

3. **Some Family Members Stress You Out.** Ration your time with them. Plan to be apart. See them in a different way. Know what to expect.

4. **Getting the Family Organized.** Some members just won't cooperate, but with modern technologies for communication and organizing, you can do better with those who will "get with the program."

5. **Divvying up Chores.** Each family member should be pulling on the oars of the boat, but some need reminding or pushing. Get it organized. Reward or punish as needed.

6. **Poor Communication (or Lack of It).** Most relationship problems, though certainly not all, arise from poor communication. Make mealtime conversation meaningful. Take a walk together. Listen actively. Speak up.

7. **Handling Arguments.** Sometimes clear communication is not enough. The two parties have different, conflicting, needs or goals. Respect each other. Look for mutually agreeable compromises. Speak your mind and listen carefully. Be willing to lose little fights if you can preserve more important values.

8. **Agreeing on Parenting Decisions.** You both love your kids and want what's best for them. Your biggest decision was whether to have children or not. Now that they are here, many issues will arise. Approach them rationally and assuming good faith in your partner.

9. **Balancing Work and Home Life.** You don't want to be Jack of "All work and no play made Jack a dull boy." On the other hand, you probably have to work to get the money you need, and you may want to work because you like your work and advancing your career. Once you've provided for the essentials, how much more to work is a matter of taste...and discussion.

10. **Staying Close-knit.** For career opportunities and for other reasons, families are often spread over the face of the Earth. There are few people who care about us; most of them are usually family members. Cherish them. Make time and space for them. If you can. Regular family meals with meaningful talk will help.

So, we find practical, rational approaches to overcoming family blockages and strife, but some of the blockages are in our own personal energy, our emotions toward our family and its history, our desires for how these relationships should progress. Getting at these problems in a non-traditional way is what my sound techniques achieve.

Family issues are one of the most common areas people see me for help. They find they have trouble achieving what they want with their most important relationships.

Renee is a woman in her mid-50s, recently divorced, with two kids. She was financially comfortable, but she felt lost.

She found my show on a telesummit.

Her voice sounded muddled.

"I thought your 30-minute package would help me. I get choked up, and my voice sounds odd, like a teenager, with my voice cracking. I want to present myself better, with a good, clear speaking voice, a confident voice. I want to be taken seriously when I speak."

I had an idea about the source of this problem. "Tell me about your family."

She said, "I grew up in a strict, religious family. I had four siblings. My folks were good providers, but they were into 'tough love.' Dad was quiet, and we children were expected to be quiet, too, especially at the dinner table. In general, we had to be prim and proper–and seen but not heard. My voice was muted, shut down."

"This problem does seem to come from your childhood experience."

"My dad was very serious, and we did not have a close father-daughter relationship. He was a blue-collar worker. When I came home from school, I was expected to do my homework or clean my room and behave myself. And when we were at the dinner table, my dad used to yell, which intimidated us, and I was frightened."

"I can tell from your voice and your story how it is that your voice has gotten suppressed. You probably had similar issues with guys you dated."

"Yes, I was attracting men who were a lot like my father, talking over me. I want to be more outspoken."

"Let's go back and imagine you are now that child at the table, and we are going to release that blocked energy. We are going down to your stomach and move that trauma energy, as you listen and breathe deeply."

I started making my sounds and observing her changing. She was crying.

"Just let the energy go, releasing it through your head as you breathe deeply."

She told me that her body started shaking. She added, "I can feel something coming from my stomach…fear…terror… energy."

I made more sounds, of different tones. I could tell she was responding.

She said, in surprise, "I can't believe I am holding all this sadness."

"Yes, you are holding years of hurt. Even though your father did not intend to hurt you, his behavior did."

I could tell she was more relaxed. I reminded her that this release would continue for several days.

"Feel different?"

"I do feel different," she said clearly and then she started coughing.

"Your throat has opened," I noted.

"Yes, I thought before that there was something wrong with my throat, but now it feels unblocked. I feel that something has changed—from my solar plexus to my heart and chest and throat. I can actually breathe more freely."

She added that she had not gotten such results with other methods she had tried.

I encouraged her, "Just remember this will continue to improve. You may or may not need another session."

We got off the phone. I was pleased, and she must have been, also.

A couple of weeks later, she called me, "I feel like a new person, much more confident, my voice is fine, and I am going to interview for a job."

Later, she wrote me a testimonial, and she repeated those same words, "I feel like a new person."

There are many causes of energy blockage, and certainly not all come from our childhoods, but often they do, because we absorb so much from how we are treated as children. Adults have to be careful. Parents bring a lot of their own issues to their parenting. Renee, as a five-year-old child, was not able to speak up in the presence of her dominating dad. Fortunately, I was able to help release the blockages that kept her from having the grown-up, confident voice she so much wanted.

Chapter 10

DISCOVER THE ULTIMATE YOU!

A BOOK LIKE Mike Hernacki's *The Ultimate Secret to Getting Absolutely Everything You Want* dares us to seek what we currently don't believe we could have, to think beyond our current boundaries, to follow the examples of many others who combined the power of the human mind with the power of the human will. Analysis and intention, reason and emotion, an open mind and a positive attitude…these can be keys to a new life.

We are told that the human brain is greatly under-used, having much more power than generally harnessed. At times, we suspect we have abilities and talents as yet untapped. This can lead to a picture of being energy-blocked, something that my sound techniques can address and often improve.

I work with groups, sometimes as large as 100. I am associated with a company in Minneapolis, Learning Strategies, which has been in business for 37 years.

Every two weeks I meet with the group, as part of a six-month course, meeting by instant teleseminar. We work on clearing different unconscious mental blocks: self-love, true happiness, expansion, passion in your life, health and well-being. This has been my third year with the organization. A new group starts in September 2018. We will be working on new themes.

In these 30-minute calls, we go into some silent clearings, having the attendees think about the topic, letting their minds wander, and examining what's not working for them. Using my sounds, I then help them release this energy. We return to listen to extra sounds while they do controlled breathing, and they find that much of their mind chatter goes away.

I start the meetings with grounding the subjects, grounding their life-force energy, getting them to be present. We clear various chakras, starting from the head and working down, unblocking their energy. Down through torso, legs, feet, to link with Mother Earth.

Then we move to another topic within the session's specific theme. Attendees are to note what is blocking them.

At the end of the session, we have a clearing sound. I end with a sound of integration, so the energy will continue to work for days to weeks after the call. The participants are to go back to their normal lives with the clearing continuing. Testimonials indicate a strong response.

As I noted, this is a six-month course; we need a real commitment, as we pursue getting to the ultimate you.

Chapter 11

Overcoming Fearful Resistance to Your Life's Mission

If you are not where you want to be, probably something is blocking your progress. Removing such blocks is one of the goals of my sound sessions. Once your obstacles are removed, you are free to progress as you wish, for example to create and run a business that you enjoy and that brings you enough money that you no longer worry about it.

Dawn (nice name!) Gluskin wrote about 7 "spiritual blocks" that can get in your way, and she gave the following advice [https://www.huffingtonpost.com/dawn-gluskin/success_b_5088207.html]:

1. Don't stop believing.
2. Fix financial woes.
3. Don't quit before the finish line.

4. Bust through internal blocks and limiting beliefs.
5. Listen to your gut.
6. Be adaptable.
7. Be in alignment.

Can my techniques help you channel your energy to do these? I think so.

"Rose" (not her name) worked with me for three 30-minute sessions. The deep information did not come out at the first session. In the first session, I usually do a general clearing of a person's energy fields, helping them come to know what their energy is and what is energy from others. This tends to make them feel more peaceful, more centered, less scattered.

"Rose" was an empathic person. After the first session, she signed up for another. A month later, we had a very interesting second session. I could detect a harshness to her voice; something was constricting it, changing it. I intuitively picked up on some of her problems.

I asked her, "What are you doing with your life now?"

She replied, "I'm happily married to my husband, and I enjoy reading to my grandkids, and I chat with my neighbors over the fence."

"Do you do anything else outside of the family? Are you working with others in the outside world?" I asked.

I could tell she was resistant. I asked much the same question again.

"Do you do anything just for fun, just to socialize with others? I think you need to be more open, more welcoming."

FEAR FREE MADE CRYSTAL CLEAR!

"I did have a passion years ago. I wrote two books and worked hard to market them, to get them sold and read. I had written them easily, but it was hard to get others to promote them."

"I think you need to put more of your energy into those books again."

"They seem too simple, and I don't think they will help others."

She had become argumentative. I needed more information.

"You should put more of your energy into them, as it is clear that you enjoyed writing them. How was your childhood? It seems to have been unstable."

She admitted to me, "Later in life, I found I had been adopted, and that I had been rotated around through various relatives during my first five years. I did not really feel loved. In fact, I felt I was in quicksand, and that I had nothing firm to hold on to."

That made it clear to me: "What is happening now is that you are clinging to your family, which was your support in your childhood, but which you could go beyond at this stage."

Rose started to cry. "I did not realize this, but you are right: I felt passed along from one person to another, and now I am afraid I will lose my family."

With my sound techniques, we did some clearing of deep emotions: of not being loved, not cared for, and not supported.

Then I told her, "Rose, you need to start again, to find something more that you care about, perhaps these children's books that you wrote."

"OK, I'll do that. Let's book another session for a month from now."

About four weeks later, we linked up with each other on the telephone, and I asked, "Hi, Rose, how are you doing?"

"Great!"

"What has been happening?" I could already tell her voice was lighter, less tense.

"I realized that I feared I would lose my immediate family, feared they would die or something. I made some calls, and I got my books picked up by someone with connections to libraries and with connections to make them ebooks." She was clearly excited.

She apologized for being so resistant in the first two sessions, and she thanked me for expanding her horizons, making her less fearful. She was very happy. We did a clearing at the end of this third session, and she had little remaining blockage.

I find that many of my clients are stuck and would really like to contribute to the world around them, but they are afraid to do so, often not knowing how to start. By removing this fear that is blocking them, and sometimes by suggesting a possible path for the to try, I have often had them expand their activities and expend their creative energies and become happier people by doing so.

Chapter 12

Clearing Self-Sabotage

What is "self-sabotage"? Using your own energy against yourself. You are misdirecting it, dangerously. Two skilled professionals (Mark Goulston, MD, and Philip Goldberg) have written an excellent book about this, *Get out of Your Own Way: Overcoming Self-Defeating Behavior*, with 40 chapters on specific things we often do that sabotage our endeavors. [https://www.amazon.com/Get-Out-Your-Own-Self-Defeating-ebook/dp/B00BWVGJY2/ref=sr_1_2?s=books&ie=UTF8&qid=1525293674&sr=1-2&keywords=self-sabotage]

The tendency to defeat ourselves interferes with much we hope to accomplish. Imagine how much better your life would be without it. Next, I tell you about a session I had with a client who had this problem.

Yesterday, Julia, a feisty lady from Louisville, Kentucky, called and had a 30-minute session with me as part of one of my packages.

Julia is now living in one little room. She was hoping to get into a new situation. She had been married to an alcoholic for 40 years, and after he died, she found he had spent all their savings, so that she now has little retirement. She is just getting by on Social Security.

What was she hoping to accomplish with our session? "I'd like to find out if I have any special talents. My world has fallen apart. I got use to having a husband who handled things, and now I am stuck in a tiny apartment, with no room to have the grandkids visit."

She was in her early sixties, with these recent problems in trying to make ends meet. She was unaware of her own abilities. Our initial session was to clear her internal energy of fear-based vibrations cluttering her system.

We did some clearing exercises.

"Julia, you are in a fight-or-flight, fearful status. To relieve these fears, I am moving your energy through your body, down through your feet, grounding you to planet Earth."

I could tell she became calmer, as her speech was smoother and slower.

I could also tell she had been lacking self-confidence. "Living forty years with an alcoholic spouse has made you co-dependent, lowered your self-esteem, and clouded your thinking. "

We cleared some pain, especially in her shoulders and lower back, where there had been much stiffness.

"Oh, my god, I feel a lot better!"

As I often do, I asked, "What was your childhood like?"

                    FEAR FREE MADE CRYSTAL CLEAR!

"My father was an alcoholic, and my mother was pretty much unavailable to me emotionally, rarely showing me love."

"That's why you looked for love from a man to replace your father. Unfortunately, you came to rely too much on this new person, weakening your own power."

We did some more sound-energy work. Clearly, she had the low energy that is typical of self-defeating thoughts.

We did another clearing, this time a deeper, silent clearing. I had her keep thinking while I removed her self-sabotaging energy. She was to think about what was not working. While she thought about what she did not like, I ran some more sounds, then I changed what I wanted from her.

"Now, stop thinking about those negative things, and listen to my sounds, releasing all the stuff you have cluttering your mental box, somewhat like the stuff you have jammed into your tiny apartment. How does that feel now?"

Her voice was transformed. "I feel so much better, not so trapped any more. The stress overload is gone."

I could tell that she needed to practice picturing what it was she wanted. "You should start journaling, centering on the things you want in your life and planning the actions needed to obtain them"

Suddenly, as though awakened, she said, "I want to get a pet! I will get a job with the humane society and start helping those animals." That was something she could do right away, not needing a larger apartment, Moreover, she would be earning some more money, while doing something that she loves.

It was a magical transformation.

A majority of the people I work with have this self-sabotage element in their thinking. I often find it comes from a childhood trauma or one from later in life; sometimes it seems obtained through the family genes. Often something will shift during our sessions, and what is in their unconscious comes out. It is amazing to me how rapidly this happens. Perhaps the energy-moving sounds allow the transformation to flow without getting bogged down in words and rationalizations. All this in thirty minutes!

Chapter 13

CLEARING LACK OF SELF-WORTH

WHEN I CHECKED with the massive online bookseller Amazon, they were offering over 5000 books on self-worth and about 500 on self-esteem. In their less-expensive, Kindle ebook listing, there were still over 1000 titles, including *How to Love Yourself* and the *Self-Esteem Workbook.* Clearly, there is lots of interest in this topic.

One of their most favorably reviewed books was somewhat of a classic, *Self-Esteem: A Proven Program of Cognitive Techniques for Assessing, Improving, and Maintaining Your Self Esteem.* Several reviewers wrote of the benefits they received from the diligent application of these analytical techniques over time, learning how to interpret your life.

Rather than using such cognitive-analytical methods, my sound-session technique works rapidly with your emotional/energy centers, often producing rapid improvements by unblocking your internal energy.

Here is an example of such a session, from yesterday.

I worked with Mary Ann, an immigrant from somewhere in Eastern Europe. She's a hard-worker, and she and her husband have been pursuing the American dream, successfully. They are well off.

She had bought one of my programs, and we talked on the telephone. Her story is rather common. Like many of my clients, she has been an over-giver. Such people are often taken advantage of. Her husband has a cable TV company, and she does lots of the office work and the paperwork.

She has raised the kids, managed the home, helped with the business. She has made no time for herself.

"Mary Ann, with all the time you put in doing things for others, do you ever get some time for yourself?"

"It never seems I have enough time to do that."

"Why are you not honoring yourself and taking care of your wants and needs, perhaps even your passions? Do you have any hobbies?"

"No hobbies."

"What was your childhood like?"

"My mom raised five kids, and my father was very busy. The pattern was tough love, if there was love at all."

"I believe you did not get much love, especially being one of five kids."

"True. I watched my mom try to get my father's approval, affection,

                    FEAR FREE MADE CRYSTAL CLEAR!

and attention, working herself to the bone. She was always nervous, always striving, always achieving. My father was grumpy when he came home, and my mother was trying to keep the peace and make everyone happy. I do think I have taken on some of her qualities. She did not seem happy. I can't remember seeing her smile. I've picked up her give-give-give pattern. I have not been happy myself."

"This is where we will start: clearing some of your belief system. Let's clear some of these. You think you have to over-give to be worthy, to feel worthy. This is a false belief."

"I'm ready to change."

"OK, picture your mom, imagine your mom. You are watching her, seeing what she is doing."

Mary Ann started to cry. I made some of my therapy sounds.

"Things are starting to get lighter for me," she said after we did some energy clearing.

Mary Ann indicated she felt helpless to do anything about herself or her mom. We did some more sound-energy clearing

"How do you feel now?"

"This heavy energy is leaving me, along with the tears. Wow! It is like a cloud that is lifting off me."

We did a lot of clearing for the thirty-minute session. She had been experiencing real feelings of unworthiness, which became resolved.

Besides the energy clearing, Mary Ann also needed some energy grounding, which I did with her.

Before we finished, I assured her, "Even after you stop with this session, the clearing will continue. Now take a couple of deep breaths. You seem to have made progress. How do you feel?"

"I feel almost giddy. A cloud has lifted. A heavy blanket is gone."

"Spend some time every week just for yourself…even schedule it on your calendar if you have to. Be sure to do something you'd like. Become a bit like a child, get the play you did not have back then."

"'I'll do that," Mary Ann affirmed. "I feel I know what direction I have to go. I'll email you in a month or so. I've tried other healers, and I have not had a breakthrough like this with them."

That was yesterday, and I am looking forward to hearing from her.

This fear of being unworthy, of not measuring up, is all too common. We all are so busy. Some feel unworthy because they have lost touch with themselves. They feel they cannot reach the levels they imagine they should. Truly, they need to take a step back and think about themselves and make time to do some things they enjoy to rejuvenate themselves, to generate pleasant energy rather than more work energy. Taking some time, like sitting in a natural, outdoor environment, can make you understand better what is working and what is not working in your life. These ideas that come to you when you are relaxed will help you make some new moves, change some directions, following your soul. I call this "soul guidance," and we need to heed it.

     FEAR FREE MADE CRYSTAL CLEAR!

Chapter 14

CLEARING YOUR FINANCIAL MESS

I'VE BEEN "RICH" and I've been "poor," and "rich" makes life easier, but our happiness need not be dependent on our finances. We need to get our finances in order and then stop worrying about them.

One good approach is "minimalism," getting rid of what is unneeded, buying only what is essential. When you are out of debt or on your way, you can loosen up a bit, but remember "waste not, want not" and "make do, do without; use it up; wear it out" and "a penny saved is a penny earned."

To go beyond minimalism, you can heed the advice of such classics as *The Millionaire Next Door* and *Rich Dad, Poor Dad* and *Think and Grow Rich*. Knowledge is power.

If fear is preventing you from changing and cleaning up your financial mess, then my sound-session techniques may help free you from this fear, allowing you to take the steps necessary to keep your financial ship afloat.

Here's an example. I find that many of my clients are in a scarcity model. You'll note some similarities between Teresa's situation and that of Mary Ann in the preceding section.

Teresa and I did a Skype session. She was calling from central Europe. In fact, many of my clients are from France and other European countries. She had bought my "abundance program." It included a 30-minute session with me.

Her English was a bit hard to understand, but she could understand me.

"What would you like to work on today?"

"Abundance. Whatever I do, the money I make just seems to evaporate, just goes away. It seems already accounted for."

Teresa is married and works as a teacher. This scarcity problem has continued for years. She'll get a bit ahead, then quickly fall behind.

"How do you feel about yourself generally?"

"Kind of depressed. I never feel very happy."

"Are you and your husband happy with each other?"

"We work together well, but the energy in this country is low and it pulls me down. I don't like the politics."

"I understand. Do you have kids?"

"Two grown children, and I'd like to retire in my sixties in a few years, but we don't have enough saved to retire."

"Your energy seems not very lively."

"Yes, that's how I always am."

"What do you do for fun?"

"We take a walk now and then, but we would really like to take a cruise. We are glad we are both healthy, but there is not much here we can do to enjoy. As a child, I grew up with five siblings. My parents worked hard, but there was not a lot of interaction with them, as they were working so much."

"Any vacations?"

"No, we did not have the money for that. There are few extras over here."

I did sense that she was an empathetic person, an empath, which is a nice personal trait, but it is a trait that makes you vulnerable to the moods of other people. Sometimes empaths build barriers to keep from feeling too strongly the emotions of others.

"I've had a protective shell around me all my life."

"You need to get rid of that, to interact with other people more openly as your real self. This will allow the universal energy to come to you. Right now, you are blocking it; you don't feel worthy to receive it."

"I understand. There was no fun, no laughter in the life I lived."

"We are going to make you feel more alive. This will help create abundance for you."

We did some energy movement work, with the divine light. I felt a heavy energy presence, from Teresa's parents. It was hard for her to get rid of this. We released the energy that was not really her. We went deeply into her ancestral energy flows, going back several generations. I would stop every minute or so to check with her.

"Do you feel energy moving?"

"Yes, I am starting to feel lighter, freed up."

"Is it OK if I clear the heavy armor you have around yourself?'

"OK."

We moved that armor away.

"I don't know what you are doing, but I do feel the heavy energy moving away."

"That's good, but I will show you how to create a lighter protective barrier, a bubble of white light. Every morning, look in the mirror and see yourself surrounded by a bubble of white light. Tell yourself that you have replaced the heavy armor with a light boundary that will keep the energy from others from depressing you. Do this daily. You will have a light shield that will allow abundance to come to you, especially in the way of insight and ideas."

I had her take some more deep breaths, and we grounded her energy and integrated it for a few minutes.

   FEAR FREE MADE CRYSTAL CLEAR!

"How are you feeling now?"

"I feel a heavy layer has come off me. I see more clearly…and my feet feel more solid, stronger."

She was excited. I invited her to start journaling about what she wants, visualizing it clearly.

I hope to hear from her within a month. She sounded so much more positive. She also sounded grateful.

I find that a lot of the people I work with all over the world have a scarcity mentality that comes from their ancestors, their parents and grandparents especially. Releasing that heavy energy helps clear their way to abundance. When people experience the release, they feel it immediately, and it continues after the call, for days and weeks, as they have told me through email or a subsequent call. They are freed from entanglement in the old energy and attitudes that have contributed to their financial problems and restricted their access to abundance.

Chapter 15

Clearing Fear of Scarcity

Some people are not in financial trouble but are scared they might be someday. In the generation that grew up during the Depression, many feared they might return to such times of scarcity. In the extreme, these fears can lead to making irrational decisions about money and even to hoarding. At the least, such fears are unpleasant.

An inexpensive and worthwhile Amazon Kindle ebook is Felicity Friedman's *LAW OF ATTRACTION: Scarcity No More: Powerful Techniques & Strategies to Develop an Abundance Mindset*. The reviewers praised it for helping them understand the "scarcity mentality" and how to escape from it.

A longer, more expensive, religiously oriented book uses the *Bible* to help its readers escaping scarcity mentality, *The God Guarantee: Finding Freedom from the Fear of Not Having Enough*. The author is Jack Alexander, recipient of the Ernst & Young National Entrepreneur of the Year Award.

Such educational resources can be of significant help. However, if you have taken prudent steps to assure adequate future income and you find that you still fear scarcity, then techniques, such as mine, that work on one's emotional energy can be of particular value.

Here's an example.

Yesterday, I worked with Odile. She bought the Abundance program. Like many of my clients, she had to deal with a scarcity mentality. We had a 30-minute session.

"Hi, Odile, what country do you live in?"

"France."

"We'll do a 30-minute Skype session."

"I love your sounds as I heard them on the telesummit. I want to work on abundance and scarcity with you. I am not receiving enough abundance, and I am experiencing scarcity."

Odile is 56, divorced, a music teacher. She barely goes from paycheck to paycheck, even though she has lots of students, especially for singing. She has much trouble saving.

"Do you like living in France?"

"Yes, but it is expensive."

I started with "checking in" to get her life story. Her divorce was within a year, a surprise, coming after five fine years of marriage. Mood swings just overtook her husband. Her parents are no longer alive.

"Let's find out why you cannot hold onto your money."

"Must be something I am doing." She was taking responsibility, a good thing.

I asked her about her childhood. Her parents were originally from another country, Hungary. When she was growing up, her parents worked, worked, worked.

"I felt we were just barely getting by. We all complained about scarcity. Mom rationed food for eight kids. My dad worked in a factory. I have taken courses about manifesting more money in my life, but they did not work."

"Yes, we have to clear your unconscious mind, clear it of ideas from your childhood. Your energy blockage is heavy. I will start making some sounds to help you release these old thoughts, these historical misconceptions."

"I should be getting more clients and making more money, rather than just getting by."

I had her imagine a light above her head, and I found a frequency that seems appropriate for her.

"Start releasing that energy from your childhood, where your mom is worrying about feeding the kids."

I sensed lots of energy was flowing from her.

"I feel like a big ball of energy is being released from my stomach. I have been feeling sick to my stomach and constipated."

      FEAR FREE MADE CRYSTAL CLEAR!

"Yes, you have been holding your energy in. You are going to release that energy." I continued making my sounds. "How are you feeling now?"

"Well, I am feeling lighter, and I am laughing…unexpectedly. I've never felt this way. My family was always so serious!"

I continued with the energy-unblocking sounds and Odile continued with her controlled breathing.

"How do you feel? Look in the mirror."

"I see someone who is looking happy, with wide-open eyes, with a big smile, which is a surprise, because I never smile and laugh like this!"

"You've just had a 'three-minute facial.' That smile indicates your soul is happy to be home." [The "three-minute facial" is an extra I give to many of my clients, and when they look in the mirror, they see a change has occurred, making them more glowing and youthful…and it stays with them.]

"I am feeling more happy, having more energy."

We did another clearing after that. We then went into a silent clearing, where she was to think of everything that is not working and is causing her not having enough abundance, while I imagined moving her energy within her, clearing her unconscious mind.

"Take some more deep breaths." She did.

"Think about all the things that you don't like about not having abundance. Take some more deep breaths. How do you feel now?"

"A big weight has been lifted, and I see more clearly, with hope. The problems of the world that were on my shoulders have been lifted."

"Odile, you are 56 years old, and your soul wants to welcome another life-partner. You will be attracting others who want you to be happy and living abundantly." I added some more sound work and grounded her at the end of the session.

"Odile, how do you feel?"

"This has been life-changing for me. I will be getting more programs from you."

Most of my clients end up wanting some abundance work. They don't realize that they have absorbed their family's opinions about scarcity. If you have children, be careful about what you tell your children and about the examples that you give them, because they are storing unconsciously the ideas of scarcity or abundance you transmit.

Chapter 16

CLEARING THE BLOCKS TO WELCOMING AND RECEIVING ABUNDANCE

RECENTLY, MUCH ATTENTION has been given to the abundance mind-set, the philosophy underlying the book and movie, *The Secret*, akin to some of the ideas in the classic book by Napoleon Hill, *Think and Grow Rich*, currently explained in a series of books by James Goi, Jr., including his highly praised *How to Attract Money Using Mind Power: A Concise Guide to Manifesting Abundance, Prosperity, Financial Success, Wealth, and Well-Being.*

To take advantage of the insights of the manifesting abundance philosophy may require some re-direction of your own emotional energy, using techniques such as mine to remove blockages.

Here's an example.

I worked with a guy two days ago, Gabriel, from Jerusalem, interacting via Skype. He had bought my abundance program, and this was our 30-minute session.

He needed more money.

"Hi, Gabriel. Amazing to be working with someone from Israel. You got my abundance program. What shall we work on?"

"I'm blocked with respect to money. I found you through the Learning Strategy program out of Minneapolis. I have had people I trusted with whom I invested, and then I lost it. Some even stole it. Money seems to fly away from me. I've been married twice. My first wife left me, and went to the United States, and then she and all our seven kids died in a fire."

"How are you coping with that?"

"I am trying to manage my emotions and to help others to cope with similar loss. I have remarried, but I do not have children by this second marriage. Moreover, I cannot seem to get financially healthy."

"I can tell there is something going on with you." I started the session. He was in a park or something, as there was so much noise. "What is that noise?"

"I'm in downtown Jerusalem."

I could tell he was troubled by the noise, lacking peace, getting much distortion from the chaos.

"You are feeling the world's energy." I could see his aura, and I cleared all his seven major chakras, down to the stomach. They had all been

     FEAR FREE MADE CRYSTAL CLEAR!

blocked. Such blockage prevents abundance. His energy field, his aura, cleared.

"How do you feel now? Do you do any energy work yourself?"

"I don't do any myself, but I am now feeling a bit lighter, less stressed."

"Do you do any meditation?"

"No, I'm too busy."

"Your heart chakra is blocked. If you open it up, you will be able to love more. You will get over not having been loved by your family as you grew up." I did some more heart chakra work, by having him envision someone who loves him and whom he loves, as I made sounds to expand the heart charka. I saw his sadness and pain leaving. He was thinking about someone he absolutely loved.

"Take a few breaths. How are you feeling?"

"Oh, my gosh, I am feeling a lot lighter, a lot better. I think I have been shut down all my life, never feeling loved. I think they did love me, but I was not feeling it."

"We have to clear that belief system that makes you think, as a male, you do not need, nor do you get love. You think it is not strong, not manly to feel emotions. Love and abundance work hand in hand."

I cleared the love blockage, one that had been propagated through the males in his family line.

"Are you willing to make yourself vulnerable?" I asked.

"Yes, I do need to be able to receive love and abundance, just as I need money to do what needs to be done."

Making a specific set of sounds, I cleared all the blockages from the past generations.

He continued to cry. "Oh, I am feeling exuberance and love, even in this short session."

"Take a deep breath. How are you now?"

"Lighter and much freer."

"Open your heart to receive love and money."

We could not clear all his energy, but I advised him to keep working on it after our session. I advised him to keep using my abundance program, which would help him to get a deeper level of clearing of his blockages. I was moving energy through his subconscious mind, and I had him think about all the reasons he did not like not having enough money. We cleared these blockages for a few minutes.

"Gabriel, stop thinking about that now. Breathe and release while I clear out the energy remaining after the last treatment. How do you feel now?"

"Oh, my gosh, I am actually feeling my heart, which is unusual. I like this feeling of an expanded heart."

"Now you are available to receive abundance. You are ready to receive as well as give."

"I feel a flow of energy from my feet to my head."

I had one more topic I wanted to be sure to cover with him. "We need to talk about boundaries…while you are in Jerusalem, imagine you are encased in a protective bubble, an energy boundary, the bubble of life, and keep it with you as you do your daily activities. Now that I have cleared out the energy that was not good for you, you will use the bubble to keep outside influences from being able to push disruptive energy into you."

He commented that he appreciated what we had done, and he told me he had received much more in the 30-minute session than what he had from just listening to the recordings. He received much more than he expected, he said. He was clearly much relieved.

Over the years of working with people, I have had many clients who have complained about not receiving abundance. Usually, this it is a heart blockage, where they did not fell worthy of receiving good things. Money or abundance comes from opening the heart chakra. I could see that Gabriel was blocked there. After our session, the universe could then bring abundance to his unblocked self. In a few weeks, he should see more abundance coming to him, as most of my clients have told me has happened to them.

Chapter 17

CLEARING FEAR OF LOSING A BELOVED PERSON OR PET

WHEN MY FIRST dog died, he was ten years old. I continued to cry for the next two and a half years.

My second dog, Hoku, now eight years old, has been with me since he was a puppy. He is almost my child, and I know I will be heartbroken when he dies. I have had so much loss in my life, I find it easy to sympathize with my clients who have experienced similar losses.

Sadly, when you fall in love, you are going to cry someday, or someone will cry over you. Death is a fact of life. Perhaps if there were no death, life would have less meaning, no challenges, as there would be no reason to do anything NOW, because an infinite time would be available. All could be postponed to *manana*, tomorrow, "soon enough for me."

We can understand death and yet fear it for ourselves and our loved ones. We can reduce that fear by thinking that there are likely to be many years before the end. We can hope they will go to heaven, or we can be thankful that their suffering has ceased. I think that life never really ends, we just go from being a material being to a spiritual being.

We can plan how we are going to handle the deaths of those we love, and we can investigate many sources of help, such as the recently published book *Good Grief: Strategies for Building Resilience and Supporting Transformation* (Barrett, 2018).

When all the intellectual approaches have been tried, and even before they all have been tried, we can harness my sound session techniques to reduce or eliminate the fear energy that has built up within us. I'll share an example of when I served as a medium to connect a client with a beloved one on the other side:

A few years ago, I did much of my work in person on Maui before I became globally known. For example, I worked with a woman in the town of Kihei. She found me from a local ad I had put in a magazine. We'll call her "Ruth."

Ruth and I met for her session at her condo. She seemed in her late 50s, thin, with a dog and married to a husband who was not there at the time. The home was a bit run-down, and the neighborhood seemed risky.

We drank water and started to talk.

"Ruth, can we have our session here now?"

"Yes. My husband is out right now."

"What would you like us to do?"

"My son passed away a few weeks ago. He lived on the Mainland, and he struggled with depression. I could not afford to visit him, as my husband controls our finances strictly. On his last call, my son, Jeff, indicated something was wrong, but he did not make it clear. I told him I would like to visit him but could not. He used to call me every few days, then the calls stopped for a week, and I got a call from the Oregon police that they had found my son shot to death, a suicide, in his bathroom.

She started crying bitterly.

"Dawn, I can't go forward. I wish I could contact my son; I wanted so much to be with him."

"Yes, Ruth, I sense that Jeff is coming through me in this session. He is telling me that it was his time to go. His words are coming through me. He wants you to know how he is feeling."

Ruth said she could feel his presence. So could I.

"He wants me to remind you of how he would wear his hat backwards on his head and tell you that his belly is still big and bouncing."

"Oh, that is something so like him, but almost no one else here knows that."

"He has dark hair, and he is a bit overweight at just under six feet tall."

"Yes! Yes!"

"What do you want to tell him, Ruth, that you could not before. Tell him now, as it is hard for me to hold him with us much longer."

"I'm so sorry I could not be with you, Jeff."

"Jeff is saying, 'Mom, I am at peace now. I have no pain. I have visited you and signaled you by dropping things on the floor to let you know I was there.' Jeff wants you to move away from this husband, his alcoholic step-father. You have to go to a battered women's shelter right away."

I could see Ruth brighten up.

"Ruth, Jeff told me you should not worry about the money. It will come."

Ruth was crying tears of joy. I made a high-pitched sound to ease Jeff's passage back to the other side.

"How are you feeling? I had no idea Jeff would show up."

"Gosh, this wholly changes my life. I feel he is with me. I understand he felt it was his time to go, and I feel much more at peace with this. I am going to get out of this situation and get a place of my own,"

I helped ground Ruth's energy, and I cleared her apartment of the low-density energy.

As we parted, Ruth said, "I feel healed. I feel like a new person. I am so grateful. I am going to take some action to get away from here and from my abusive husband."

She scheduled a session with me for a month later. This one we held in a local beach park. We sat on the grass together. I did not bring her son to her, but I did bring her some guidance. She had the good news for me that she had found some people who help abused women, and she got a new place in another town not too far away. She said she was amazed at how her life had been transformed so much and so quickly. She felt glad that she had trusted me for the sessions. She felt her son was now going to continue to be a part of her life.

I think that it is always good to know that, as spiritual beings, we are connected with others deeply. When we love a person or a pet, the spiritual connection is never broken. They are always a part of our lives, here or on the other side. Life continues, either physically or spiritually. Our loved ones are looking at us with love, compassion, and support, even when they are on the other side. Knowing this should help us enjoy our lives more and not fear death. This is the cycle of life. Life does not end. It transforms.

Chapter 18

Clearing Fear of
Your Own Death

"**Everyone wants to** go to heaven, but no one wants to die," an anonymous wit is credited with saying. Yet, die we will, eventually. We will find out the truth about the Afterlife then. Meanwhile, we may worry. Ideally, we will take the prudent steps needed to improve our chances at long life and try to live each day aware that it might be our last. Our fear may make us careful or it may distract us and thus risk a premature ending.

When I searched amazon.com for books about fear, I got over 40,000 titles. It's a big issue for many of us. A recent book, *Curing the Dread of Death*, goes into the topic in great, helpful detail, as explained by psychologists.

Fear can make our days unpleasant, wasting what life we are granted. Fortunately, my sound-session techniques can help relieve this fear, making your days more pleasant, fear-free. You can be as free of fear as you are when sleeping. You will not be like the joker who described life as "the somewhat-less-pleasant period between naps."

Here's an example of how I addressed one client's fear of death:

This was a child, "Danny." It was a while ago. Few children come to me, but this was one, a special case.

Danny was a teenager, about 14, and his mother had done a session with me. He had two siblings. The family was stable, but he has had this issue since he was five or six, when he became unusually afraid of storms. The parents had him see MDs, but nothing was clearly wrong. A psychiatrist could not figure out why he could not sleep without having the lights on.

This was Danny's first energy-healer experience.

"Will you work with me for 30 minutes and be open to the possibility it may help?"

"Yes, my mom says that what I am doing is unusual."

"Do you have problems at school?"

"Yes, I am sleepier than I think I should be, and the doctors say that I am not sleeping well enough."

"I am going to make sounds and check on you and see how you are doing. I see that the family seems fine, and you have good relationships with your brother and sister."

"Right."

                    FEAR FREE MADE CRYSTAL CLEAR!

"I am bringing some energy to you to see what is in your unconscious mind."

"That's fine. I've tried doctors, and I still need the lights on."

"Imagine a divine light right over your head. Breathe deeply." He was breathing shallowly, from the very beginning. This is not very uncommon.

"Do you notice that you are not breathing deeply?"

"Doctors have told me that, but we don't want me to take drugs, like Xanax, for anxiety. When I do go to sleep, I often wake in a cold sweat."

"I'm not a doctor, but we'll work on what we can to try to improve your sleep. I see something in your energy. You may have had a past life when you were someone very different. You seem to have been a soldier in a war, perhaps the Civil War. Do you know any history about the War?"

"Yes, I am very interested in that subject, and I have a natural tendency to study it. I have had some dreams in the past about being on a battlefield."

"Could it be in Gettysburg?"

"Funny, my family took me there once. I saw the re-enactment when I was about eight. I started crying."

"Yes, Danny, this is what I am picking up from you. Can you believe you might have lived before?"

"My mother is open to that, and I'll think about it."

We started the clearing process, and I had him imagine he is on a battlefield. "You were there and lost your life."

He started crying after I made my sounds. He said it was hurting him, as he was dying.

"Keep releasing the energy that is coming through you."

"It is amazing. I don't know where this energy is coming from, but it seems from my stomach up. It is amazing."

Then he quieted.

I told Danny, "Keep breathing deeply. The energy is being released from your past life. Take a couple of very deep breaths. You are releasing the energy from your past life. Open your eyes."

"Oh, my God, I can tell I am breathing better, and the world now looks much clearer, and I feel much at peace, no longer sad."

We were nearing the end of the session.

"Danny, I want your mom to email me in a few days, to tell me whether this helps you to sleep better."

"Yes, my parents were amazed I knew so much when we visited Gettysburg."

A few days later, his mother, Elizabeth, wrote that the session including the past life was so effective. Later, I learned that he slept the first week with the lights on, but then the second week without them. "He has really changed, and this is the only solution we have found," she wrote.

FEAR FREE MADE CRYSTAL CLEAR!

I replied, "Our souls live on. He is now cleared of this trauma. He should no longer be troubled by it."

"That's a miracle. Thank you so much. That was so good!"

That was about eight years ago. It was one of the most significant transformations I achieved. The imagination of this child, the continuation of his soul, reassures me that we live on in another form. There is not a beginning or end to our spiritual being. This session let him move forward with his life and be in better health. It opened Danny to new possibilities in his life.

Chapter 19

CLEARING FEAR OF BEING SEEN

A MORBID FEAR of being seen or noticed is "scopophobia." Sometimes it is associated with schizophrenia, but in milder forms it is akin to stage fright.

The Conversation, a 1974 American movie starring Gene Hackman, dealt with a surveillance expert who eventually became afraid that he himself was under continuous observation. He goes to extremes to keep his conversations private, but he fears he cannot do so. The movie ends with his mental breakdown.

Few of us have such extreme fears, but the milder forms can be troubling. Fortunately, I have found that my sound-session techniques can be effective in reducing such fear.

Here is an example.

Let's call her "Phoebe." She heard one of my telesummits and bought a package that included a 30-minute intro session. She lives on the East Coast and is in her 60s. She sought abundance for her life.

"Hi, Phoebe. What would you like to work on?"

"I'd like to work on abundance. I am on Social Security."

"I'll scan your energy. Are you married? Kids?"

"No, I've been alone by myself all my life, and that is how I like it. I do things like listening to these telesummits."

I could tell she was spending much money this way. Too much?

"Have you had a relationship with someone you love?"

"No, I had a few relationships that quickly ended up with being abused, taken advantage of. I do love my pets."

"What do you do all day?"

"I stay home and listen to programs, including these telesummits. I do a bit of gardening, too."

"Do you have a social group, like a seniors' group?"

"No."

Her life sounded something like how my own had been at one time.

"How did your parents treat you as you grew up?"

"They sheltered me, treated me as someone too different to be seen by other people. I never felt love from them. They seemed ashamed of me."

"That seems the problem. How were you so different that your parents wanted to hide you?'

"I would say stuff that people did not expect, such as predicting a relative would die. My parents were uncomfortable with such predictions and talk. They would shush me and put me away. I told a neighbor her dog would die, and it did so soon thereafter."

"I can understand that people did not feel comfortable with this. Your throat is raspy, and we can work on that. You can become a new person, even in your late 60s. Working together, we can do it. I am a mover and shaker of people who need to change their lives."

"Yes, something told me to buy your program. You seemed right for me."

"Now this lack of love in childhood is showing up in your 60s. You are afraid of being yourself."

I detected a kind of shield or barrier around her.

"We need to clear this barrier you have surrounding you. You need an open heart to receive this. Are you ready for us to tear down this wall created when you were a child?"

"I'm ready."

"Imagine a light above your head. Think about that childhood incident in the store, where you predicted the dog's death as a six-year-old. Allow all that to pass out of your body and into the light."

"Yes, I felt so ashamed after that."

"Let's clear that."

She started crying deeply, very deeply.

"That old story is holding you back. We are releasing it. Breathe deeply and release."

Her crying stopped. I cleared her throat chakra, and when she spoke, I heard her voice more clearly.

"The embarrassment your parents felt was then transferred to you, and we are going to clear it, and we will forgive them for their mistakenly doing this."

She named some relatives, friends, and former boyfriends to be forgiven.

"I feel we have crashed that wall. I'm feeling numb. I have not cried in 25 years. I am glad I could do it today."

Because she indicated she needs to get out, I reinforced this. "Since you are 68, you should now go out, even seek a part-time job, perhaps with animals."

"Yes, I do want to go out."

I told her to journal about her new life. "Sit down, write, as soon as you can, about how you want your life to be. What do you want? Whom are you seeking? Open yourself to these possibilities."

We did some more sound-clearing, including heart activation. I brought energy from her childhood all the way through to her present self. After the heart activation, I grounded her.

"How are you feeling? Take a few deep breaths"

"I feel free! I never felt this free before. I feel love. I feel like a new person. I am very grateful for your work, Dawn, and I am going to follow your advice and find a way to help animals. I am ready to change and to take action. I am glad to understand why I was afraid to be seen by others."

She kind of reminded me of myself. I had felt alone and not understood. I was by myself, without a reliable friend, someone whom I let in and who let me in. I was an outcast, which made growing up so hard for me. I was never included in the popular group. I have found that it does not have to remain that way until you die. I was a hermit for 15 years, and I have gotten over it. I was my own mentor, through my soul, my heart, from which has come my sound-energy gift.

If you are determined to be happy and be more sociable, you can do it. You can become a new person, as I did. I am now received warmly by people from all over the world, and especially by those who have had hard lives themselves.

Don't you give up. A better life is possible!

Chapter 20

◇◇◇

SUMMING UP

I STILL HAVE some battles that I must wage to help me overcome what traumas I went through in my earlier years, battles which make me quite attuned to similar problems that my clients bring to me. My past brings me an occasional upheaval that I must work through.

I used to deal with these upsets by becoming numb. Now, I channel my inner energy to help me cope. I no longer need Xanax, which tended to suppress the emotions rather than clear them up.

The current drug/opioid crisis is related to this, as people are taking drugs to deal with physical and emotional pain. We need a better way to handle these pains and fears.

I do feel that to be an authentic healer, one needs to have gone through the hardships and come out at the end with wisdom. I've come from Hell and returned with knowledge, not with empty hands.

I hope that all who read this book get its major lessons: there is hope; there are cures; you are not alone; triumph is possible. We do the best we can.

One source of inspiration is the Serenity Prayer of Alcoholics Anonymous, written by American theologian Reinhold Niebuhr:

God, grant me the **serenity** to accept the things I cannot change,

Courage to change the things I can,

And **wisdom** to know the difference.

[Emphases added.]

The traumas of your life can be transformed into opportunities for strengthening you, and when you heal, the healed, scarred regions are even stronger.

There are reasons why you went through your struggles, and you can rise from them, like the legendary Phoenix re-born from the ashes, to have a new and better life for yourself and to share with those you know and love.

FEAR FREE MADE CRYSTAL CLEAR!

Testimonials

[These include some testimonials also presented in *PAIN FREE*. These are not limited to the reduction of fear, and they have had minor editing, primarily to preserve the privacy of their writers.]

Hi Dawn,

I am in such deep gratitude to you and your amazing work

I contacted you to work with my beloved dog and not only did he receive healing, I also got an amazing session with you

You are a truly divine being and for anyone that is looking for healing... Dawn is an incredible healer...

Lots of love and gratitude

N

Dear Dawn,

I purchased all your energy downloads and have been playing them regularly since summer and I must say, they make me feel at peace and full of optimism. We also had two one on one session which I enjoyed immensely. My life has become more of experiencing trust and lightness which I am so very grateful for. You certainly have helped lifting much burden from my shoulders. Thank you so very much for your immense support!

May the light guide you at all times, always, much love

C

Part of me felt kind of stupid and crazy for signing up for this even though I've been using your programs for decades. I mean, I can't exactly afford it, and it's just some lady making weird noises over the phone. But my intuition kept urging me, so I went for it.

I'm almost 50 but had such an excruciating childhood, I've still suffered the effects no matter how hard I've tried everything under the sun to heal. Some things have helped but not enough to quell the constant underlying desire to end it. I thought about killing myself all the time as a kid, and the desire always remained no matter how hard I tried to heal and think positive. I would never do it because I wouldn't leave my child alone in the world, and I knew it was just leftover darkness, but to varying degrees it was the backdrop to even the happiest of times for my entire life.

                                        FEAR FREE MADE CRYSTAL CLEAR!

Well, yesterday was Suicide prevention day, and I realized that I had not thought about killing myself for several days. That weight is gone. There's light in that place. So, that's pretty cool for only one session. Thanks for that. I'm excited to see what happens next.

L

Dear Dawn,

Being an energy healer, medical intuitive, empath, animal communicator myself, I can truly say that you are very gifted and that your sound healing frequencies are very strong and effective.

I thoroughly enjoyed the private session you so generously included in the purchase of your total body Rejuvenation program. It made me feel so much better, more grounded and alive. But most important I could feel your passion for your work. You truly want to be of service and your heart connection with the client is very strong. It has been an honor connecting with you via Skype.

Thank you 🙏 you are an inspiration for me.

With Angel blessings,

A

August was a particularly difficult month for me. Fortunately, I had my private session with Dawn on September 3rd. That session was phenomenal. I released much negative energy I didn't even know I had. That night, I had the first good night's sleep I have had in a long time. The dreams were positive, too, instead of ones about some tragedy or another that I had to overcome. I am currently working my way through the series of Abundance Blocks mp3's that were part of the package I bought and find them helpful as well. My energy is now more positive, and I wake up looking forward to how the day will unfold instead of thinking this is just another day I have to get through. Dawn is truly amazing. I connected with her energy during the webinar she was on and the connection became more evident when I spoke to her on the phone. You will not regret purchasing any of the packages she offers as she is sincere in wanting to help you and not just wanting to make a buck pushing a product you really don't need. She helps you find the true you that is part of the Whole/God. Once you find that part of you and learn how to allow what your desires to manifest instead of resisting those things you are attracting that you don't want, you will find your life has changed forever in a very, very positive way. I am truly grateful I found the one person who could get through my resistance and help me birth the part of me that is truly part of Source/God. Now I can continue exploring what is mine to do in this lifetime allowing only those energies that are in my highest good to manifest themselves in Divine timing. Dawn helped me, and she can help you, too, if you choose to allow that to happen.

D

I was in extreme pain back in the latter part of June/July. I do not know where it came from and why, and my appointment with Dawn was scheduled for July 21. I asked Dawn if she could move me up or squeeze me in because I was experiencing excruciating pain that I had

                    FEAR FREE MADE CRYSTAL CLEAR!

never felt before. Since someone had rescheduled, she had an opening for the July 7, and I was able to take that spot. Dawn did what she does best with her sound healings and going to the core of the problem, I didn't even notice, but my pain went away and that next week, the pain was gone. It went as mysteriously as it came. It was miraculous. Thank you, Dawn, so much for your generosity and flexibility.

J

Dawn,

You're a magical gift to my life. Finding you randomly one evening after being guided in a dream by my grandfather who I channel with often, he gave me a perfect description of the person who I needed for my next healing. That very next day in my inbox I received an email that had a re-play of one of your online talks, I knew immediately seeing your picture you where the exact person my grandfather had described the night be-fore so I proceeded to listen to your free healing followed by purchasing the get out of pain package which included a private session with you. As I proceeded to schedule my first solo appointment with you I was able to book my appointment the very next day which once again I knew this had to be more than divine intervention. My first solo appointment I noticed immediate shifts in my life so much I paid for a second solo ses-sion. I can't thank you enough for sharing your gifts with the world, your generosity at the end of my second session with a free bonus extra healing but more importantly releasing blocks that have hindered me for years.

You're a true blessing,

L

Thank you so much for the information, Dawn. Today, I woke in a different world with a more positive attitude. You hit the nail on the head with the resisting. Unfortunately, allowing is easier said than done. I allow for infinite possibilities for infinite flow/abundance/happiness in my life every day when I do my chi machine exercise. I have been doing this for several months and I am still waiting. The resistance may be part of the shields I put up years ago when I felt I needed them to protect myself from verbal abuse, etc. Recently, I have been working on lowering those shields even though that leaves me vulnerable again. I am going to presume my subconscious does not want to let them go. I will work with more of the mp3's that you included in your offer. I know if I am persistent enough, eventually everything will work the way it is supposed to work.

Thank you again for the wonderful session yesterday.

Namaste' and aloha,

D.

Dawn, hi, it's Y****, the last caller from Monday's show. I wanted to write a testimonial and since I couldn't find where to submit it, I thought that I'd just send it to you here: Thank you, thank you, thank you! Those few minutes working with you changed my life completely! Especially in relationships. But most importantly, I finally feel

  FEAR FREE MADE CRYSTAL CLEAR!

the self-love that I couldn't before. I, for the first time in my life, feel deserving of love.

Thanks again, Much love and blessings to you,

- Y.

Hi Dawn, I was the one who was suicidal the other night when you were on Spaced Out Radio with Elizabeth Anglin. It took a little while, but as the night went on, I progressively felt better, and I wanted to thank you for that.

- L. M.

I am listening to the Live show right now....and I Feel Fabulous! Thank-You, Thank-You, Thank-You, Dawn Crystal....Many Blessings to you for the Awesome work you do!!!

- D. R.

Dawn, I am in rediscovery. The stranger that was my lost self returned to me by your powerful energy work. I feel clear-headed, balanced, grounded and in total amazement of the self I have to get acquainted with. I am ready for the new world that is coming at us with great speed--and your energy work makes me fearless of whatever the future may hold.

With heartfelt gratitude, and love,

- I.

Hi, Dawn, I had the honor to get selected tonight for you to work with me. I am S., living in ****, NC. I have to admit that when you started in with your sound healing, I said 'What!' I removed my judgment and just went with it. When you selected me for a brief session, I wasn't sure what to expect. While you were working on me, I felt light-headed. After a while, I started to feel lighter and more joyful.

Thank you!

- S.

Hi Darius,

I don't have an intention for this week. Instead, I just wanted to tell you that I bought a package that included a personal session with Dawn Crystal and it is the best thing I have ever done! To put it in a nutshell, I can't even remember why I wanted to work with her. (This is a good thing!). I found a list this morning of things I had wanted to address

                    FEAR FREE MADE CRYSTAL CLEAR!

with her and was shocked that I had felt those things (fear, depression, etc.). **They are just gone**. Anyway, I hope you have her back. She is a true blessing.

By the way, if you use any part of this note for your show, please do not use the name on this email. You can call me Liz from ****** if you need to say anything. (No last name please)

Thanks, LP

Hi, Dawn, thanks so much for the session earlier I feel much lighter already and am looking to clear even more. I'm always so appreciated for your healing. It's really a blessing that you are providing this healing to the world. :)

- A.

I am so Grateful to have had my issues addressed...I slept so good...and I have had a very rough 4 months... Thank You to Dawn Crystal for assisting me....I felt so much calmer after the session...just knowing I was helped in some way

- K.

I appreciate hearing your story that you shared on Lauren's show. I just listened to the replay & the healing I felt was Amazing!!!Your courage to follow your inner guidance is deeply inspiring.

- C. A. H.

Dear Dawn, thank you so very much for the session yesterday. It was right on the money, and I really appreciate everything you did to clear me. I am feeling much lighter, and you really pinpointed some issues for me. I look forward to working with you again.

Take care.

- J.

Hello Dawn, this is J., the first caller on Monday's show. Wow, what an intense session that was!

My body was a rocking and rolling and releasing so much!

I feel like I'm still processing, and I haven't been feeling well (anxious, etc.).

Thank you so much!

- J.

The winter depression has also lessened, and I was able to attend a family function that for years I had not gone to this time of year, and as well, my energy levels are up, which isn't usual for this time of year.

- A.

Hi Dawn, First of all, I have to tell you I absolutely love the work you do and the results I get. I am part of the Learning Strategies Tues. eve. group.

You have been such a blessing in my life. In fact, I listened to last Tuesday's event again early this morning. I know I will sleep well afterward....

C.

Hi Dawn! I wanted to thank you for the healing tonight on Lauren's call! I feel so amazing! I did buy your Higher Self package and I have a session with you this Saturday. I did have a question in the interim; I know you mentioned healing abundance was part of one of the benefits of this package. I was also interested in your Wealth package too.

C.

Hi Dawn,

Wanted to let you know, following my session, this past Sunday, April 15th, I did keep focusing on letting stuff release and integrating higher frequencies. Feelings/emotions did come up and Tuesday evening I got shown and released at a deeper level than ever before an incident with my Dad when I was about 11 yrs that was still impacting me in a very limiting way. I immediately felt more energized, and more capable of 'doing life', creating what I love and desire; shifting from a "I can't" to a "I can" come from/attitude. YAY!!!

And as you said might happen, I did feel some aches/pains in my body following the session, however, that is subsiding. :-)

Thank you sooo much!

And I look forward to our next session at the end of the month!

Love,

L

Hello Dawn,

Delighted to write a testimonial for you:

FEAR FREE MADE CRYSTAL CLEAR!

So many of us work between struggle and hope in our lives. I've been trying to manage anxiety, heal from physical ailments, while also wanting to grow into more abundance and higher energetic integrity. I have found Dawn's voice guidance and acoustic clearings to be enormously helpful and transformative. With dedication, I listen to her modules daily and also regularly journal. In only two weeks, I feel more attuned, expanded and wholly rooted in my own two feet.

Wishing you ever greater circles of influence, and much love,

A

Dawn,

'I've been meaning to send you this testimonial for a few days now but a funny thing has happened. I keep forgetting to write it because I keep forgetting I had any problems. (LOL) I only remembered now because I saw the list I had written before our session that said things like, "I am gripped by fear" or "I feel like my soul has been crushed". I looked at that list this morning and thought, "I was?"... "It did?" I can't even relate to that anymore.

It's taken a minute, but I finally understand why that is. Somehow in that session, it was as if I stepped through a thin veil into a slightly different version of me. It happened so easily and gently that I hardly noticed. The issues associated with the 'other me' have just fallen away and it feels like I have always been the way I am now. I know that sounds totally weird but who cares! I *love* the 'new' me!

I am so incredibly grateful for this transformation and the session. I don't think I have ever felt so 'seen'. To say you have changed my life for the better would be a meager understatement. Thank you, thank you, thank you!!

DP

PS - I also sent a note to ****** to let him know how great it was to work with you.

All the best,

D****

I have purchased three of Dawn's programs and had a session with her. I cannot encourage anyone enough to participate in her wonderful healing love and beautiful vibrations. I felt so much energy and love from Source through her, I was floating. Speaking with her, I felt as I was talking to my long-lost sister. She is a beautiful wonderful, truly loving lady. I am grateful that she shares her beautiful gift with us. I am grateful she has helped me remove my blocks.

Many Blessings,

S.

I have purchased 2 of your packages-Total Body Rejuvenation and Anti-Aging, both from the Eram show, and I think they are brilliant!

I think your work is outstanding and I have done much spiritual and energetic work. Thank you for your pure openness and generosity of spirit!

Much love and light,

M.

Dear Dawn,

Thank you so much for sharing your amazing gifts with me. I am so grateful for your time & effort during my 3 sessions (FHTY - Anti-Aging Package). You are truly one of a kind. Last night's final call session was amazing and releasing the soul (baby) back to Source was so right. He/she would have been attached to me for more than 26 yrs. Finally, now back with Source.

Much Love & with Gratitude,

W

Dawn,

I've tried quite a few different packages from different healers.

Your Anti-aging MP3s are amazing!

When I am listening to them I can feel energy buzzing all around my body, especially at the top of my head.

After listening I feel out of space at the beginning, but later I feel more grounded. I sleep better, I feel better. I feel connected!

Your work is very important and much appreciated.

Much Aloha!

And Blessings!

T

Hello Dawn,

The Anti-aging program works wonders! Mostly all the wrinkles on my face have disappeared and I look ten years younger. I am still working on the perfect weight part, my cravings are less, and I'm eating more fruits and vegetables. My skin is now very soft, and I am glowing. I feel totally different. Thank you Dawn for being who you are today and for helping people, as we all deeply appreciate your work! Thank you so very much!!

C. M.

[Most entries edited for privacy, punctuation, and format.]

LINKS TO DAWN CRYSTAL RECORDINGS

Healing MP3 page
https://dawncrystalmaui.clickfunnels.com/squeeze-page

HEAL ADRENAL FATIQUE & BURNOUT
http://static.wixstatic.com/mp3/14f4a3_cca37fcfbf194e-
f08ab3826c85371366.mp3?dn=HEAL+ADRENAL+FATIQUE+&
+BURNOUT.mp3

HEALTHY THYROID ACTIVATION
http://static.wixstatic.com/mp3/14f4a3_7d9ba4d1443742e6a3db96
39d3f9cd89.mp3?dn=HEALTHY+THYROID+ACTIVATION.mp3

WEIGHT LOSS MADE EASY!!!
http://static.wixstatic.com/mp3/14f4a3_32b6a30cabb44622
858a82e25b84ae35.mp3?dn=WEIGHT+LOSS+MADE+EA
SY%21%21%21.mp3

HAPPY HORMONES ACTIVATION
http://static.wixstatic.com/mp3/14f4a3_7d3083eae81c4130a27bdd
54fcfeced8.mp3?dn=HAPPY+HORMONES+ACTIVATION.mp3

HEALTHY GUT ACTIVATION (FREEDOM FROM DIGESTION ISSUES)
http://static.wixstatic.com/mp3/14f4a3_6575476411644d55926e56d5a27aa5da.mp3?dn=HEALTHY+GUT+ACTIVATION+%28FREEDOM+FROM+DIGESTION+ISSUES%29.mp3

ENERGY SYSTEM REBOOT! (RE-ENERGIZE & ALIGN YOUR ENERGY)
http://static.wixstatic.com/mp3/14f4a3_e8f-4737fe02c4b878827d567392dbd83.mp3?dn=ENEGY+SYSTEM+REBOOT%21%28RE-ENERGIZE+&+ALIGN+YOUR+ENERGY+SYSTEMS%29.mp3

LIVER CLEANSE & DETOX (DEEP HEALING & RENEWAL)
http://static.wixstatic.com/mp3/14f4a3_115c72702e8c4a5a8351bfb1fc6d035a.mp3?dn=LIVER+CLEANSE+&+DETOX+%28DEEP+HEALING+&+RENEWAL%29.mp3

STRESS BE GONE!!! (A DIVINE ENERGY CLEANSING)
http://static.wixstatic.com/mp3/14f4a3_83a2cce86b024f1f9650e58b9f61a46c.mp3?dn=STRESS+BE+GONE%21%21%21+%28A+DIVINE+ENERGY+CLEANSING%29.mp3

ALLERGY FREE!!!
http://static.wixstatic.com/mp3/14f4a3_5c7fa5a5bddd4be5a313ad7b18fa45c4.mp3?dn=ALLERGY+FREE%21%21%21.mp3

CHAKRA CLEARING & BALANCING (FOR PERFECT HEALTH!)
http://static.wixstatic.com/mp3/14f4a3_ca6abca802e4474084b-192ac6afff90d.mp3?dn=CHAKRA+CLEARING+&+BALANCING+%28FOR+PERFECT+HEALTH%21%29.mp3

    FEAR FREE MADE CRYSTAL CLEAR!

HEART LOVE ACTIVATION (OPEN UP TO RECEIVE MORE!!!)
http://static.wixstatic.com/mp3/14f4a3_dc95e9e0dfd94b-
fea40f4c96255201db.mp3?dn=HEART+LOVE+ACTIVATION+%
28+OPEN+UP+TO+RECEIVE+MORE%21%21%21%29.mp3

KICK-A-HABIT ACTIVITATION
http://static.wixstatic.com/mp3/14f4a3_7a1319ba08e84a77b803cf2
20141b560.mp3?dn=KICK-A-HABIT+ACTIVITATION.mp3

FACE LIFT & EYE LIFT (INCLUDES THE NECK AREA)
http://static.wixstatic.com/mp3/14f4a3_1549829c89234d64917ff3
00d5b2948b.mp3?dn=FACE+LIFT+&+EYE+LIFT+%28INCLUD
ES+THE+NECK+AREA%29.mp3

About the Author

Dawn Crystal, an internationally recognized Voice Sound Healer, Body-mind Intuitive, respected Intuitive Life Coach, Soul Reader, Medium, Pain Release Expert and Best-selling Author (*PAIN FREE Made Crystal Clear!*), is known as a **LEADING TRANSFORMATIONAL EXPERT** incorporating ancient wisdom for modern day success.

Dawn is passionate about helping people clear emotional and physical blockages, so they can manifest from their higher selves, step into their full potential, and lead their lives and businesses in ways that align effectively with their souls' purpose.

Dawn helps her clients to release themselves quickly from pain, emotional and physical, and she is an active mentor for entrepreneurs, CEO's, and celebrities, helping everyone! Dawn is the "go-to" person to get out of pain fast, in minutes!

Dawn participates regularly on global teleseminars, radio shows and podcasts. Dawn was recently interviewed by the *Today Show, Dr. Oz, Rachel Ray, The View*, etc. For the past few years, Dawn has done a live bi-weekly program at Learning Strategies Corporation called "Sound Healing / Silent Clearings."

Dawn's unique sound healing CD has been purchased by clients around the globe, and she is available on both phone and Skype, as well as for teleseminars.

Dawn lives a peaceful life on Maui, along with her adorable dog, Hoku.

Dawn recently published her first book in this series, *PAIN FREE Crystal Clear!*, published by Outskirts Press, available in paperback and ebook formats from Outskirts and from Amazon (amazon.com) and Barnes & Noble (bn.com).

"I wouldn't change anything about my life; it's a gift," she affirms, and she transmits this inner strength to those she works with, giving them a grounding, a stable psychological place abounding with safety and love.

"I wouldn't do it over again, but I am glad where I ended up."

To see a ten-minute interview video with Dawn Crystal, go to

https://tinyurl.com/ybg3osgp .

REFERENCES

Barrett, C. (2018), *Good Grief: Strategies for Building Resilience and Supporting Transformation.* Outskirts Press, Parker, CO, and Amazon. com.

de Becker, G. (2010), *The Gift of Fear*, Amazon Digital Services LLC.

GluskinL, D. https://www.huffingtonpost.com/dawn-gluskin/success_b_5088207.html

Goldberg, M., and Goldberg, P. https://www.amazon.com/Get-Out-Your-Own-Self-Defeating-ebook/dp/B00BWVGJY2/ref=sr_1_2?s=books&ie=UTF8&qid=1525293674&sr=1-2&keywords=self-sabotage

Green, A. https://www.mindbodygreen.com/articles/5-things-to-do-if-youre-feeling-stuck-in-life

Kondo, M. *The Life-Changing Magic of Tidying up: The Japanese Art of Decluttering and Organizing.* Ten Speed Press, Random House, 2014.

McGuinness, M. https://99u.adobe.com/articles/14347/are-you-subconsciously-afraid-of-success

Pinola, M. https://lifehacker.com/
top-10-family-issues-you-can-overcome-1674901208

Menzies, R.E, Menzies, R.G., and Iverach, L., Eds. (2018), *Curing the Dread of Death: Theory, Research, and Practice.* Australian Academic Press. Amazon.com.

Review *Fear Free?*

Reviews on sites such as amazon.com help connect readers and authors. We would appreciate it if you would write a review, even a short one.